Waterbirth Stories

Drawing on years of midwifery experience of waterbirth, this collection of stories, based on real-life events, illuminates a rewarding way of birth and emphasises the theoretical knowledge, skills, understanding, and resilience needed to practice well.

Waterbirth Stories includes chapters on the criteria for use of water in labour and birth, on the different stages of labour, and on some more serious or unusual situations such as shoulder dystocia, postpartum haemorrhage, breech presentation, and other unexpected maternal and neonatal events. Each chapter includes several stories from a midwife's perspective, told in the context of evidence-based guidelines available for this topic. The stories end with learning points to help readers reflect on their own practice.

Ideal for student and practising midwives with an interest in waterbirth, this research-informed book is enjoyable, challenging, and informative.

Maria Paz Miranda is a midwife working at an NHS Alongside Midwifery-Led Unit in the UK.

Sian Marie Barnard is a midwife working at an NHS Alongside Midwifery-Led Unit in the UK.

Waterbirth Stories

Midwifery Reflections

Edited by Maria Paz Miranda and Sian Marie Barnard

Foreword by Laura and Russell Brand

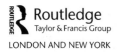
Routledge
Taylor & Francis Group

LONDON AND NEW YORK

First published 2020
by Routledge
2 Park Square, Milton Park, Abingdon, Oxon OX14 4RN

and by Routledge
52 Vanderbilt Avenue, New York, NY 10017

Routledge is an imprint of the Taylor & Francis Group, an informa business

British Library Cataloguing-in-Publication Data
A catalogue record for this book is available from the British Library

Library of Congress Cataloging-in-Publication Data
A catalog record has been requested for this book

ISBN: 978-1-138-54153-5 (hbk)
ISBN: 978-1-138-54154-2 (pbk)
ISBN: 978-1-351-01077-1 (ebk)

Typeset in Times New Roman
by Deanta Global Publishing Services, Chennai, India

I would like to commend Maria Paz for conceiving the idea of writing this book and thank her for inviting me along on this literary journey.

Sian Marie Barnard

Contents

Contributors

Catriona Cusick is a midwife working at an NHS Alongside Midwifery-Led Unit in the UK.

Pat Hutson is a midwife working at an NHS Alongside Midwifery-Led Unit in the UK.

Foreword

Our waterbirths

Laura and Russell Brand

Both of our daughters were born in a birth pool. Both of our daughters arrived, calmly blinking into the light. No tears, no screams. Two completely unique labours but one constant. Water.

I had read a lot of books, spoken to a lot of people, and watched an abundance of positive birth videos online when I was pregnant for the first time, with Mabel. It hadn't started off this way, however. I didn't know what to expect; it was all too easy to be distracted by fearful birth stories or filmic references. Drama, swearing, and things not going to plan. I had a couple of friends, however, who had experienced incredible waterbirths. I would ask them to recount these stories, aghast and intrigued by the recurring factor that the water had somehow made this life-changing bodily experience not only seem manageable but also otherworldly. As though the water had acted as a portal to another dimension, a place you go to collect your baby calmly, safely, and return to start a chapter new. With the encouragement of Russell and my growing belief that I could experience something quite unique, I decided to commit to understanding in advance the process of labour: what I might feel, how I should manage the sensations, and what options I'd have along the way. I met some incredible women, who guided me and educated me. Catriona Cusick was one of those women. She visited me when I was unwell with a gastric bug at 35 weeks. I was staying in the Maternity Unit on the same floor as the Spires Birth Centre, which she runs smoothly, efficiently, and calmly within the John Radcliffe Hospital. She suggested a book I should read on mindful birthing and had the kindly, unflappable certainty that as a new mother you require from people in authority. She assured me at a time when I could have easily lost the confidence that would be essential in the weeks to come.

It was around 11 a.m. on 4 November 2016 when Russell and I arrived at the Spires. Despite the previous rehearsed trips here, an 'expectant parents tour' (bizarrely, one father asked a long litany of questions but exclusively about parking), the gastric bug admission … everything felt very different, warped, and surreal. I don't have much recollection of heading to the seventh floor as I clung to my pillow, pausing to bury my face as a contraction came and went. We had practised hypnobirthing in preparation for today, so Russell pulled out the typed-up techniques and reminders (that I had laminated – ever hopeful of their use around water!) and prompted me as and when adrenalin or fear crept in, as they do, to come between you and serene nature. When we called the birth centre from home, my main priority had been to ensure we told them we wanted a birth pool. Water has always been my friend for aches and pains, so I was keen to experience the remedial effects it is known to have during labour as well. Maria, who I will come to adore as another midwife warrior, issues the disappointing news that I am only 3 cm dilated and that I will have to wait in a pool-less antechamber. At this point I was struggling; I felt claustrophobic and hot and my mind was trying to take over. A few hours in here, continual showers and a few breathing exercises later, I was finally reaching further into the labour. As I went into this more animalistic state, our beloved midwife Maria ushered us through to a small, dark room with a glowing birth pool and psychedelic lights. This was to be my happy place. It was the difference for me between day and night. I got into the pool and I felt the sharp intensity of before dissipating into a swirling warmth of the now-deepening surges. It felt like I had tumbled into a cocoon the moment I got into the pool. I was able to connect with my body's purpose as hours went by unnoticed (although that could have been the gas and air), the water soothing me and keeping me light on my toes as I got into my ultimate birthing position. I was squatting, eyes closed, facing Russell and holding onto him for dear life, or dear life-force, channelling additional energy into this momentary circle of creation, and Mabel whooshed into the water like a cosy little bullet. I could hear the echo of Maria telling me to pick my baby up and as I looked down, I could see this peaceful being floating there, waiting to be lifted, waiting to be loved. In my arms, her eyes still closed, silence – I would have panicked if it weren't for the quiet smiles surrounding me. Then just like that, her eyes opened, and she looked at me and I told her, 'Hello. I am your Mummy and you've done so, so well'.

After the birth of Mabel, I felt grateful. Grateful that I had a healthy baby and that Russell had been such an active birth partner but also that I was able to experience such an incredible waterbirth in a safe and supportive environment.

When I was pregnant with our second daughter, Peggy, I was unsure if I would be able to get close to that magical feeling once more. I started to think it may have been a 'one off' and in the final weeks of my second pregnancy I became quite fearful of what it might be like this time around. At 41 weeks and five days, on 22 June 2018, Russell was on the phone to the Spires again, letting them know that my labour had begun. Things started very slowly that morning; I was having gentle contractions far apart and so we decided to go for a walk. It was one of the many gloriously hot days of the summer and the contractions gained a little momentum as we walked through the heat. We were almost home, my waters released, in the middle of a field, and with relief and excitement, we headed off to the Birth Centre. Unlike my first labour, this journey was calm, only breaking from chitter chatter with Russell to breathe through each contraction. When we arrived at the Spires this time, we were expecting to be told we'd have a long wait ahead of us. The room was different – light, airy; the pool was larger; there were birthing balls and a single bed. I was unpacking and settling in when Catriona came to check on me. I wanted an examination, because I wanted to know what was in store. To everyone's surprise, I was 5 cm. Catriona told me there was a pocket of water that was yet to break, but that once this had released, our baby could be born quickly. I could see that the birth pool was being filled – a bit early? I thought. It was around 3:30 p.m. I hopped off the bed and as if an unseen weight was pulling me downward, I dropped to the floor in an intense wave of what I now know was established labour. I couldn't open my eyes. I kept them closed, breathing deeply into the surge. Russell encouraged me towards the pool and I was helped into the warm, welcoming water by the midwives. It hardly needs to be stated that birth is a female process and in this gentle and encouraging coven, I imagine that I am not by a birthing pool but among rocks in a beautiful lagoon, being held by women, being held by water. Once I was submerged, I felt the urge to push. Russell intuited my concerns about pushing. During my labour with Mabel, I had wanted to push for hours yet been advised that I wasn't ready. I was thankful for my husband understanding me on this level right now. So, with no words necessary, he confirmed with Catriona that I should indeed push. It was intense; there was no time for gas and air. Catriona whispered that I should focus on Russell's hand. His hand? I reached for it to my left, searching for his contact. A push! The final waters release. I return to his hand again, feeling the skin, tracing it as best I can with my fingers. Another push! Our daughter's head is out. Now, tightening my grip. Eyes closed and diving inward, an almighty roar emerges from my depths and at 4:30 p.m., another little person is gently launched into the warm and welcoming world. Another little girl, another little water baby.

Acknowledgements

We dedicate this book to the women who have given us the opportunity to be caregivers during their waterbirth journeys. Through these rich experiences, we have been able to collate an anthology of anecdotal stories in which real-life events are fictionally recreated and retold. While this book draws on experiences from the authors' own practice, names and some details have been changed to protect the confidentiality of the women and their families. We are profoundly grateful to these women, whose preference for using water during labour and birth has enabled reflection and insight into this aspect of clinical practice. We believe the knowledge and guidance we are able to share as a result of such reflection will be helpful to future generations of midwives, mothers, and families.

Introduction

Maria Paz Miranda

Thirteen years ago, when I started working as a midwife in the UK, I had to open myself to the possibility of learning many new things, and having graduated in another country in the 1980s, the concept of maternal choice in midwifery was one of those new things for me to learn.

The years have passed, and I still enjoy helping pregnant women make their own choices when it comes to labour and birth. It was one afternoon, during a day off, at the house of a colleague and friend when I first realised it. We were doing it again. We were reproducing that ancient midwife tradition of telling stories, sharing our positive experiences at work, asking for advice on what had challenged our individual practice, and learning from each other's unique clinical experience. 'We could be helping more midwives and students, by writing these stories down', I thought. My colleagues did not need too much encouragement. 'Ok, let's do it', they said to my suggestion. That is how the idea of this book was born.

And here we find ourselves, committing our experiences as midwives to pen and paper, compiling them into a small book. In fact, the four of us have accumulated more than 36 years of clinical work in the last nine years, helping women labouring and birthing their babies in water, and more than 70 years of midwifery experience altogether. We practice in an alongside NHS midwifery-led unit, under the umbrella of NICE and statutory bodies' guidelines, where the use of water in labour and birth is a popular resource readily available to help women in their wonderful journey into motherhood.

In the first chapter, you will find a brief and basic introduction to midwifery in the UK and its changes through the decades. The second part of the first chapter addresses the criteria for the use of water in labour and birth in the UK, as it is defined in the clinical guidelines currently available in the country.

In the second and third chapters, we go on to share with you our experiences of the latent phase of labour and established labour respectively, both entities probably being the most difficult and complex diagnoses for a midwife to make. You will find examples where, by using water, we were able to reduce obstetric intervention and help women during this intricate transitional journey, from the latent phase to established labour, to finally achieve a successful spontaneous vaginal birth, resulting in high levels of maternal satisfaction and safety.

The fourth and fifth chapters describe two of the most common obstetric emergencies encountered by midwives independently of the birth setting: postpartum haemorrhage and shoulder dystocia. We share how we have faced these situations with women in the water, including the step-by-step management of these situations and the resulting outcomes.

The sixth chapter is dedicated to those unexpected situations that took us by surprise, putting our professional skills and responses to the test. We would like to believe that our ability to overcome these emergencies is due to our capacity to work together, as an articulated team, that has helped us to deal with these unexpected events. At the end of each chapter, we share our reflections to encourage discussion and learning.

We sincerely hope that the stories compiled in this book, in which real-life events are fictionally recreated and retold, and the identity of women protected, will help midwives and students, especially those who are newly qualified and are looking for clinical orientation in a field that demands theoretical knowledge, practical experience, and resilience.

Chapter 1

Use of water in midwifery in the UK

Maria Paz Miranda, Sian Marie Barnard, Catriona Cusick, and Pat Hutson

Introduction

The provision of maternity care has changed dramatically over the last few decades across the planet, with, sadly, wide differences in its improvement according to the political, financial, and educational resources available in each country. Nevertheless, globally, the maternity death rate has decreased thanks, amongst other reasons, to the incorporation to the midwifery practice of better training, new drugs, and the formulation and implementation of clinical guidelines.

In this first chapter, we would like to introduce you first to the particularities of midwifery and maternity care in the UK, its evolution throughout the years, and the incorporation, in the last few decades, of the concept of 'maternal choice', which includes the use of water in labour and birth, within the wider context of the National Health Service (NHS). To be able to fully comprehend the relevance of the previous statement, it is important to remember some of the key principles of the NHS since its creation in 1948:

- The NHS provides a comprehensive service, available to all.
- Access to NHS services is based on clinical need, not an individual's ability to pay.
- The NHS is accountable to the public, communities, and patients that it serves (Department of Health and Social Care, 2015).

As midwives working in an NHS maternity unit in the UK, we work under these principles. We believe that the implementation of maternal choice within maternity services, specifically in the case of 'place and mode of labour and birth', has been made possible, amongst other reasons, because of these key principles mentioned earlier. In this context, we believe that respecting and promoting maternal choice, which includes the use of water in labour and birth as one of the pain-relief options available, is essential in achieving a high level of safety and increased levels of maternal satisfaction, whilst still adhering to statutory bodies' guidelines.

The second part of this first chapter is dedicated to the description of a basic criterion for the use of water in labour and birth throughout the country, with samples from different hospitals and National Institute for Health and Care Excellence (NICE) guidelines.

We sincerely hope you enjoy reading this first chapter. We would like to believe that it provides the reader with the necessary basic historical context to comprehend our stories and where they have come from. Also, the stories provide an insight into how far we have come, in terms of being able to facilitate maternal choice during childbirth.

The birth of midwifery within the NHS: Catriona Cusick

In the early nineteenth century and before the NHS was founded, maternity care was mainly provided by midwives. They attended childbearing women at home and worked independently from the medical profession. These midwives were untrained, unregulated, and often unpaid; the skills and knowledge they acquired would usually be passed on from veteran midwives to their inexperienced counterparts.

Infant and maternal deaths were high due to factors such as poor nutrition, inadequate sanitary conditions, and the lack of maternity provision (Reid, 1990). Doctors were not legally obliged to attend labouring women and this, coupled with a lack of interest and guaranteed payment, meant there was a reluctance from them to attend births when midwives were an available and free resource.

The beginning of the twentieth century saw a radical change in midwifery provision. The Parliamentary Midwives Act of 1902 was introduced to regulate and improve standards of care. As a result, the very first federal registered midwives were commissioned. The Central Midwives Board (CMB) was also formed as a part of the Midwives Act 1902 to monitor and approve training. The CMB created rules of practice that enabled continuing professional standards and registration to a legally recognised regulatory body (Arney & Neill, 1982). This altered the person present at births from the lay practitioner or handywoman to the registered midwife. With the introduction of the Midwives Act 1902 and registration as a prerequisite, midwifery became the domain of educated women, and therefore, the ownership of midwifery practice was transferred from the unqualified layperson to an erudite body of women.

Most women at this time were still having homebirths, but thanks to the Midwives Act, they were now mainly attended by registered midwives. Any woman who practised midwifery unregistered was fined if caught; however, caring for women in labour was still seen as an additional income rather than a professional occupation. To monitor adherence to necessary regulatory stipulations, local authorities started to pay midwives a salary and a pension to improve enrolment. This improvement in standards also meant that pain relief was made available to childbearing women at home, whilst still having the process of normal, physiological birth supported.

The next major change that brought an improvement in maternity service provision came with the birth of the NHS. Its foundations were based on the work of the economist William Beveridge and the coal miner Nye Bevan, who pursued their political aspirations to become leading figures in the drive to improve the health of the nation. Beveridge compiled a report in 1942 in which he recommended that the government should find ways of fighting the five '"giant evils" of Want, Disease, Ignorance, Squalor and Idleness' (Beveridge, 1942). At this time, the country was in the grip of the Second World War and Beveridge identified the poor general health of the soldiers as being attributable to limited access to quality healthcare. However, the key recommendation of his report was that he felt it was 'imperative to give first place in social expenditure to the care of childhood and to the safeguarding of maternity', stating that the 'health of the nation' was dependent on the health of maternity services (Beveridge, 1942).

In support of this incentive, the Labour prime minister of the time, Clement Attlee, acted as the catalyst to the introduction of the 'Welfare State' as outlined in the recommendations of the Beveridge Report (Beveridge, 1942). In 1945, Attlee appointed Aneurin Bevan as the Minister of Health, affording him the responsibility of instituting a new and comprehensive National Health Service. Bevan's own humble background shaped his political intent; as the son of a coal miner, Bevan was driven by a desire to address social inequality. He became a champion for social justice, fighting for the rights of working people. In his role as Minister of Health he was perfectly placed to spearhead the establishment of a health system that would be accessible to all, regardless of wealth. Both Attlee and Bevan had the foresight and passion to realise that the health of the nation was paramount to the future of the country.

In support of this sentiment, a public campaign was launched. Women played a big part in this campaign and were fundamental in helping to raise awareness about the inequality in healthcare provision; they literally swung the vote and became known as the 'silent majority'. As a result, in just six months, on 5 July 1948, the NHS was born – an inclusive national health service with no fees and that was free to all. The following years brought changes to the political establishment and a change of prime minister. In 1951, the Conservative Party succeeded Attlee's Labour government and Winston Churchill (previously in office from 1939 to 1945) returned to power for a second time. Both Churchill and the British Medical Association were opposed to Bevan's ethics; they were a formidable force and a real threat to Bevan and his ideals of an NHS. Bevan fought on though, stating that 'no society can legitimately call itself civilised if a sick person is denied medical aid because of lack of means' (Bevan, 1952).

This was literally life-changing for those who had not previously been able to access quality healthcare. Doctors, midwives, nurses, dentists, and other practitioners specialising in a wide variety of disciplines were employed by the NHS to run the service. The service was funded by the working population's tax contributions known as National Insurance.

The NHS incorporated and retained the Midwives Act of 1902 within the NHS Act of 1946 but appointed local health authorities as the supervising authorities in place over midwives instead of the local councils. They had to exercise general supervision over midwives practising within the area and to investigate allegations of malpractice, neglect, and misconduct.

By the mid-1950s, confusion arose over how much the provision of the NHS was costing and an inquiry and review into maternity services were called for by the government of the day (Davis, 2013). The Earl of Cranbrook was appointed to lead this investigation, resulting in the 1959 Report of the Maternity Services Committee, otherwise known as The Cranbrook Report of 1959. In this report, a target for 70% of all births to take place in hospital was recommended with the committee deciding that the remaining 30% of mothers could safely give birth at home. The midwifery profession was being shaped by regulations and governmental committees, which meant that the growing control of hospitals and physicians was starting to define maternity care in categories of safety and risk.

John Peel, an obstetrician and gynaecologist, headed several steering groups, committees, and government agencies. He went on to instigate a report in which the provision for all women to labour and birth in a hospital setting, regardless of background, became a reality (Peel, 1970). So, it was at this point that community care and homebirths were greatly reduced, and maternity care shifted into a hospital environment. NHS midwifery services were divided between hospitals, GPs, and local authority health services which included antenatal clinics (Davis, 2013). This meant a fundamental change for the place of birth and where and how midwives practised (McIntosh & Hunter, 2014).

In opposition to this, several maternity pressure groups such as the Natural Childbirth Trust (NCT, 2009) and the Association for Improvements in the Maternity Services (AIMS, 2018) argued that most women did not need to be in hospital to give birth safely. The reactions of the NCT and AIMS pressure groups combined with the many, ceaseless campaigns led by advocates for normal birth meant that maternity care within the NHS would continue to be scrutinised in order that the importance of individualised care would not be ignored. The feminist movement and groups such as the Association of Radical Midwives also had a voice regarding women's rights. These movements postulated the concept of autonomy within midwifery, encouraging midwives to empower women by supporting their choices (Kitzinger, 2006). The concept of having fathers and families present at births also reinforced the philosophy of giving the ownership of birth back to women. The concepts of choice, control, and continuity of care or carer were now the overriding issues in the provision of maternity care (Winterton, 1992). The impact that social and psychological factors have on pregnant women and their families was acknowledged, and women were being encouraged to make decisions about their antenatal care and birth (Beech, 2009). New standards for maternity care were also highlighted in 'Maternity Matters' (DOH, 2007), in which attention was paid to personalised choice, the choice of midwifery care, and place of birth. Several surveys conducted at the time revealed that most women did not know they had a choice of where to birth, or that home birth was even an option. Concerns regarding a lack of information for women regarding their choices were also highlighted by surveys conducted by the National Perinatal Epidemiology

Unit (NPEU, 2010), the Care Quality Commission (CQC, 2010), and the National Audit Office (NAO, 2013).

The Birthplace Study (NPEU, 2010) looked at perinatal and maternal outcomes by planned place of birth for healthy women with low-risk pregnancies. Findings showed that midwifery units appeared to be a safe option for both mother and baby. It was noted that there was no significant difference in the incidence of adverse perinatal outcomes compared with planned births in hospital. In addition, a key finding was that women had significantly fewer interventions and more physiological births than women under obstetric-led care. In the UK, the Winterton Report (Winterton, 1992) and the Changing Childbirth Report (DOH, 1993) were pivotal in acknowledging that women should be given choice of the position they birth in and also that the use of water during labour and birth should be an available option. In recognition of this, the popularity of freestanding midwifery-led units (FMLUs) and alongside midwifery-led units (AMLUs) grew. The FMLUs and AMLUs were created to respond to the demands of personalised choice and place of birth. As part of this philosophy of care, birthing pools became an available resource during the 1990s.

We are now in the twenty-first century where most women in the UK continue to birth in hospital. However, in line with Bevan's vision of an 'all-inclusive health system that meets the needs of the nation', FMLUs and AMLUs aim to provide a safe, supportive, 'home from home' environment (NPEU, 2010). This makes them an increasingly popular choice with women whose preference is for little or no intervention during their childbirth experience. In this context, FMLUs and AMLUs offer the use of water as an extremely useful and highly valued tool that accommodates maternal choice and provides an effective, non-invasive, and evidence-based form of pain relief.

Criteria for the use of water in labour and birth in the UK: Pat Hutson

Hydrotherapy has been used in medicine for many thousands of years, with records of Roman soldiers using bathing in spring water as a form of relaxation after battles, as well as it being used as a relieving remedy for rheumatism and other ailments (Cluett & Burns 2009). It was not until the 16th and 17th centuries that hydrotherapy became scientifically understood and accepted for musculoskeletal conditions, although there are still many unanswered questions as to how water is beneficial in medicine (Tubergen & Linden, 2002). The first recorded waterbirth occurred in France in the early 1800s (Balaskas, 1996). Years later, Frédrérick Leboyer, a French obstetrician, introduced the idea of bathing babies in water after delivery. He argued that this could help to minimise the distress of birth on the newborn infant (Leboyer, 1979) (Balaskas, 1996). Leboyer was interested in making the transition from intrauterine to extrauterine life as natural as possible because he believed this could influence a baby's future life (Leboyer, 1979). Leboyer had many critics but in the 1970s Michael Odent, a former Leboyer disciple, introduced birthing pools in the French unit in which he was working at the time (Balaskas, 1996; Walsh, 2012). However, it was assumed that this 'new age' approach to birth would die a natural death within a short period of time (Odent, 1996).

In favour of the use of water in midwifery, we could say that in water the body's weight is reduced by around 75%; this liberates a heavily pregnant woman to become more mobile, thus enabling the woman to assume a more comfortable position for labour and delivery (Alfirevic & Gould, 2006). This can also influence the diameter of the pelvis, allowing the foetal head to adopt an optimal position to aid rotation and descent (Henderson et al., 2014; Alfirevic & Gould, 2006). It is also thought that immersion in warm water during labour and birth can improve the effectiveness of the contractions, optimising oxygenation of the uterine muscle and increasing venous return and mobilisation of extravascular fluid (AAP, 2014). The calming effect of the water also allows the natural hormones needed for labour and birth to be released.

It was not until the 1980s that the use of water for analgesia in childbirth was introduced in the UK (Harding et al., 2012). This was implemented due to the publication of the Winterton Report (House of Commons: Health Committee, 1992) and the Department of Health's Changing Childbirth Report (Department of Health, 1993), which recommended that women, after discussion with healthcare professionals, should be encouraged to make an informed choice of how and where they wish to birth their babies (DOH, 1993; House of Commons: Health Committee, 1992). As a result, MLUs and AMLUs, most of them equipped with birthing pools, were created in response to the recognition of the importance of maternal choice during childbirth. The appropriate set of guidelines were born and shaped to ensure a safe environment for both women and babies choosing to use water during labour and birth (Harding et al., 2012; NICE, 2017; Alfirevic & Gould, 2006).

Points to consider when caring for a woman who has chosen to labour and birth her baby in water

To ensure hygiene and infection control, scrupulous cleaning and maintaining of the pool and equipment is needed (Harding et al., 2012; Alfirevic & Gould, 2006).

Caring for a labouring woman in water can be challenging to the midwife if she/he has worked mainly in an obstetric setting (Flint, 1996). Midwives involved in caring for women using water in labour and birth must reshape their approach to natural progression in labour whilst being mindful of the need for intervention when any deviation occurs (Walsh, 2012). It is an individual midwife's responsibility to ensure they have the adequate training to be confident and competent in supporting a woman who wishes to labour and birth in the water (Alfirevic & Gould, 2006; Harding et al., 2012).

As with all aspects of midwifery, documentation of discussions of water immersion with the labouring woman should be clearly recorded (Alfirevic & Gould, 2006).

During immersion in water, the temperature of both the mother and the water should be checked on an hourly basis and, whilst ensuring the woman's comfort, the water temperature should be kept below 37.5°C (NICE, 2017).

It is not recommended for a woman who has received opioids to enter the pool for at least two hours after administration of the drug, or if she still feels under the effects of it (NICE, 2017).

Entonox can be used in conjunction with the pool to good effect (Harding et al., 2012; NICE, 2017).

There is no evidence to suggest that water immersion should be limited in time, nor is there a specific point in labour that water immersion is optimal (Harding et al., 2012; Alfirevic & Gould, 2006), although mobilisation in early labour is recommended (Alfirevic & Gould, 2006).

A baby born in the relaxation of the water often does not immediately cry and can take longer to 'pink up' (Flint, 1996; Walsh, 2012).

Once the baby has been born in the water, it is brought slowly and gently to the surface. Special care is advised in order to avoid excessive tension on the cord and potential damage to it (Garland 2011).

Each maternity unit has its own criteria for labouring and delivering in a mid-wifery-led unit, where the use of water during labour and birth is part of the pain-relief options based on maternal choice. The following list is a combination of criteria obtained from NHS hospitals in Nottingham, Salisbury, Shrewsbury, and Telford, along with NICE guidelines (NICE, 2017; Ross, 2018; Howard, 2018; Women and Children's Care Group, 2014).

Criteria for the use of water in labour and birth

- 37–42 weeks of gestation.
- BMI between 18 and 40.
- Cephalic presentation (some hospitals will facilitate labouring in water with a breech presentation; Ellaway & Hedditch, 2016).
- Established labour – cervical dilatation > 5 cm (WHO states that it could be 6 cm; NICE states it is 4 cm).
- Women expecting their first to fourth baby inclusive.
- Hb over 90 g/l.
- Low-risk medical history.
- Maternal age < 18 years or > 40 years.
- Platelets over $100 \times 10^9/l$.
- Singleton pregnancy.

Exclusion criteria (this is not exhaustive)

- (Some) known foetal abnormalities.
- History of maternal seizures.
- Known blood-borne viruses, i.e. HIV, active herpes, Hep B.
- Known intrauterine growth retardation (IUGR).
- Previous third- or fourth-degree tear.

- Previous caesarean section.
- Previous PPH > 1000 ml, or that required treatment with blood products.
- Severe immobility (individual assessment may be needed to ensure woman can vacate the pool quickly in an emergency).
- Significant presence of meconium in the amniotic fluid.
- The need for oxytocin to induce labour.

Immersion in water for labour and birth is a difficult subject to research due to the nature of the matter. Around the world, water is now being widely accepted as a safe environment for a labouring woman as part of the pain-relief options available. However, delivering a baby in water remains controversial in some countries. In the UK, the main statutory bodies and governmental organisations safeguarding childbirth, such as the RCM, RCOG, and NICE, have formulated a frame of guidelines that enable us to provide safe care. These are based on the concept of women's choices around childbirth and they allow us to help women who, after an informed discussion, have chosen to labour and birth their babies in water.

References

AAP, American Academy of Paediatrics, 2014. [Online] Available at: http://pediatrics. aappublications.org/content/pediatrics/133/4/758.full.pdf [Accessed 11 November 2018].

AIMS, 2018. AIMS for a better birth. [Online] Available at: www.aims.org.uk [Accessed 9 September 2018].

Alfirevic, Z. & Gould, D., 2006. Royal College of Obstetricians and Gynaecologists and Royal College of Midwives Joint Statement No. 1. [Online] Available at: http://activebirthpools.com/wpcontent/uploads/2014/05/RCOG-waterbirth.pdf [Accessed 29 September 2018].

Arney, W. R. & Neill, J., 1982. The location of pain in childbirth: natural childbirth and the transformation of obstetrics. [Online] Available at: https://doi.org/1011/j.1467-9566.1982.tb00245.x [Accessed 18 October 2018].

Balaskas, J., 1996. Why do women want a birth pool? In: Beech, B., ed. *Water Birth Unplugged.* Cheshire: Midwives Press, pp. 6–13.

Beech, B., 2009. Midwifery – Running down the drain. [Online] Available at: www.aims.org.uk/journal/item/ [Accessed 18 October 2018].

Bevan, A., 1952. *Place of Fear.* London: Heinemann Ltd.

Beveridge, W., 1942. *The Beveridge Report Social Insurance and Allied Services.* London: HMSO.

Cluett, E. & Burns, E. 2009. Immersion in water in labour and birth. [Online] Available at: www.cochranelibrary.com/cdsr/doi/10.1002/14651858.CD000111.pub4/epdf/full [Accessed 12 December 2018].

CQC, 2010. Essential standards of quality and safety. [Online] Available at: www.cqc.org.uk/sites/default/files/documents [Accessed 15 July 2018].

Davis, A., 2013. Choice, policy and practice in maternity care since 1948. [Online] Available at: www.historyandpolicy.org/policy-papers/papers/choice-policy-and-practice-in-maternity [Accessed 18 October 2018].

Department of Health and Social Care, 2015. [Online] Available at: https://assets. publishing.service.gov.uk/government/uploads/system/uploads/attachment_data/ file/480482/NHS_Constitution_WEB.pdf [Accessed 15 November 2018].

DOH, 1993. *Changing Childbirth – Report of the Expert Maternity Group*. London: HMSO.

DOH, 2007. *Maternity Matters: Choice, Access and Continuity of Care in a Safe Service*. London: HMSO.

Ellaway, P. & Hedditch, A., 2016. My baby is breech. [Online] Available at: www.ouh. nhs.uk/patient-guide/leaflets/files/12975Pbreech.pdf [Accessed 21 October 2018].

Flint, C., 1996. Water birth and the role of the midwife. In: Beech, B., ed. *Water Birth Unplugged*. Cheshire: Midwives Press, pp. 60–62.

Garland, D., 2011. Breathing. In: *Revisiting Waterbirth an Attitude to Care*. Basingstoke: Palgrave Macmillan, 126.

Harding, C., Munro, J., & Jokinen, M., 2012. Immersion in water for labour and birth – Evidence based guidelines for Midwifery-led care in labour. [Online] Available at: www. rcm.org.uk/sites/default/files/Immersion%20in%20Water%20%20for%20Labour% 20and%20Birth_0.pdf [Accessed 13 October 2018].

Henderson, J., Burns, E. E., Regalia, A. L., Casarico, G., Boulton, M. G., & Smith, L. A., 2014. Labouring women who used birthing pool in obstetric units in Italy: prospective observational study. *BMC*, 14, 17.

House of Commons: Health Committee, 1992. *Maternity Services: Volume 1*. London: HMSO.

Howard, S., 2018. Underwater labour and birth. [Online] Available at: www.icid.salisbury. nhs.uk/ClinicalManagement/MaternityNeonatal/Pages/UnderwaterLabourandBirth. aspx [Accessed 17 October 2018].

Kitzinger, S., 2006. *Birth Crisis*. Abingdon: Routledge.

Leboyer, F., 1979. *Birth Without Violence*, 6th edition. Norwich: Fletcher & Son Ltd.

McIntosh, T. D. & Hunter, B., 2014. 'Unfinished business'? Reflections on changing childbirth 20 years on. *Midwifery*, 30(3), 279–281.

NAO, 2013. Maternity services in England. [Online] Available at: www.nao.org.uk/report/ maternity-services-England [Accessed 15 December 2017].

NCT, 2009. Location, location, location. Making choice of place of birth a reality. [Online] Available at: wwwnct.org.uk [Accessed 15 December 2017].

NICE, 2017. Intrapartum care for healthy women and babies. NICE Guidelines [CG190] Pain relief Stategies. [Online] Available at: https://www.nice.org.uk/guidance/cg 190/chapter/Recommendations#pain-relief-in-labour-nonregional [Accessed 4 March 2018].

NPEU, 2010. The birthplace cohort study. [Online] Available at: www.npeu.ox.ac.uk/ birthplace/results [Accessed 2 October 2018].

Odent, M., 1996. Are we marine chimps? In: Beech, B., ed. *Water Birth Unplugged*. Cheshire: Midwives Press, pp. 14–17.

Peel, J., 1970. *The Peel Report*. London: HMSO.

Reid, A. J., 1990. Maternal mortality: Preventing the tragedy in developing countries. [Online] Available at: www.ncbi.nlm.nih.gov/pmd/articles/PMC2280328 [Accessed 18 October 2018].

Ross, J., 2018. Water immersion during labour and birth. [Online] Available at: www.nuh. nhs.uk/download.cfm?doc=docm93jijm4n1064 [Accessed 14 October 2018].

Rowe, R., 2017. Nuffield Department of Population Health. [Online] Available at: https://www.npeu.ox.ac.uk/research/ukmidss-320 [Accessed 18 September 2018].

Tubergen, A. & Linden, S., 2002. A brief history of spa therapy. *BMJ*, 61(3), 273–275.

Walsh, D., 2012. *Evidence and Skills for Normal Labour and Birth – A Guide for Midwives*, 2nd edition. London and New York: Routledge.

Winterton, N., 1992. *House of Commons Health Committee, Second Report*, Maternity Services. London: HMSO.

Women and Children's Care Group, 2014. Water, labour and birth. [Online] Available at: www.sath.nhs.uk/wp-content/uploads/2016/09/Waterbirth-New-Template-3.10.14.pdf [Accessed 14 October 2018].

Chapter 2

The latent phase of labour and the water

Maria Paz Miranda, Sian Marie Barnard, Catriona Cusick, and Pat Hutson

Introduction

The definition of the latent phase of labour:

> A period of time, not necessarily continuous, when there are painful contractions and there is some cervical change including cervical effacement and dilatation up to 4 cm.
>
> (NICE, 2017c)

Diagnosis of the latent phase of labour is probably one of the most challenging aspects of our clinical practice as midwives. Experience, exposition to the phenomena, practice, and even a high degree of skill does not guarantee that midwives will always know whether the woman that they have in front of them is in the latent phase of labour or the first stage of labour.

Some midwives would be inclined to admit any woman whose cervix is found to be 4 cm dilated to hospital for intrapartum care as the sole indication of the first stage of labour. Some midwives will send the same woman home, to rest, eat, and await events. What is the right thing to do? Not an easy question to answer. However, midwifery support is the key.

When we receive a phone call from a woman requesting our advice regarding the long hours that she has been contracting at home, we are presented with a great opportunity to bond with this woman in pain, to discuss her anxieties and fears, and to obtain as much information as we can to be able to help her. It is the opportunity to plan with her and her partner, instead of telling her what to do and how to do it; this is a wonderful opportunity to discuss uncertainty. As we see it, the latent phase of labour is basically, uncertainty (RCM, 2012a).

A conversation over the phone regarding the latent phase is the chance to share information, to educate the couple about what to expect regarding labour. We believe that a frank, informative, and creative conversation over the phone is a wonderful opportunity to help these women safely navigate the uncertainty of the latent phase (RCM, 2012a).

In the extremely common cases where a woman in the latent phase has been admitted to hospital, the natural process of labour changes. Once she is an inpatient, the potential risk of obstetric intervention increases (RCM, 2012a). We diminish her independence and the opportunity for her to establish her labour of her own accord (Steele, 1995). How we approach this complex situation can make a world of difference to the overall outcome. Midwives need to work very hard to keep these women within normal parameters. We believe in being very proactive, encouraging our women to consider varied coping strategies such as warm baths, massages, breathing exercises (NICE, 2017c), light eating, gentle walks within the safety of the hospital grounds, and even after discussion, the option of returning home for a few hours (NICE, 2017c).

In summary, as previously mentioned, the diagnosis of established labour can be intricate in certain circumstances. Sometimes, anxiety and fear might hinder a woman's ability to navigate the transition from the latent phase into established labour. Immersion in warm water during the latent phase can help, reducing anxiety and fear, and facilitating progress in labour. We are aware that it is a difficult decision to make. Following our instincts, applying our knowledge and engaging in open discussion with our colleagues will enable us to reach the best decision with regard to this aspect of care (Cluett & Burns, 2009).

In these four stories, the reader will find how we've successfully managed to help these women achieve established labour and spontaneous vaginal birth, using a lot of hard work, creativity, flexibility, patience, and, of course, the mighty pool!

The power of the pool! Sian Marie Barnard

Mary phoned our unit to ask for advice. She had been having painful, irregular contractions for the last 24 hours. She was 41 weeks into an uncomplicated first pregnancy and was now experiencing with what she described as very strong but irregular period type pains that were radiating round into her lower back. Mary's membranes were intact and she reported the baby had been moving well. She sounded calm but told me she felt very tired because her contractions had kept her awake all night. I reassured her that what she had experienced was normal in the latent phase and we discussed early labour coping strategies that would help her to rest and relax (RCM, 2012a). By the end of our conversation, both she and I were happy for her to remain at home. Four hours later, Mary phoned again, this time she was more distressed. She reported that her contractions had become more painful, but irregular. Prolonged latent phase was on the horizon and I was determined to help Mary to beat it with the power of water.

Whilst Mary was talking to me, her contractions were stopping her mid-sentence. She was having to concentrate on a slow, controlled breathing technique and was a little out of breath after the contraction had passed; she was working harder now. Mary had told me her story. She thought she was in labour and I wanted her to feel I was taking that seriously; on this basis, I invited her in for an assessment.

When she arrived, her contractions were quite short lasting (about 20 to 30 seconds duration and mild to moderate on palpation). I explained to Mary that because of this, my feeling was that she was not in established labour and therefore it was unnecessary for me to perform a vaginal examination at this time (NICE, 2017a). She listened, paused to think about what I said, but then asked to be examined anyway, telling me that she 'just wanted to know what was happening'.

I found her cervix to be 1 cm dilated, 1 cm long, and posterior – the station of the baby's head was −2 to the ischial spines and the baby was in a left occipital posterior position (Sweet, 1997). Mary was disappointed – she felt she had been working so hard and couldn't understand why she wasn't further along in her labour. We had another long discussion about the latent phase and about the physiology of what was happening during this time (Stables, 2001b). I also explained the significance of forward leaning and all fours positions that would help the baby's back to rotate forwards (Sweet, 1997). I shared the information with her in a positive way, putting emphasis on the fact that she was coping brilliantly. I wanted Mary to know that everything was fine. She left, confident in the knowledge that home was the best place for her to rest and re-energise (NCT, 2018).

Mary called again later that afternoon. She told me that when she got home, her contractions had spaced right out enabling her to have a doze, but that now they had come back again and were longer and stronger than before. During our conversation, I sensed her anguish and could hear she was finding it hard to cope with the intensity of the pain; so, I invited her back to the unit. My feelings were that I would admit Mary (even if still in latent phase) to formulate a plan of care that would best suit her needs. It was obvious from her call that she wanted more direct support.

On her arrival, I could see she was more distressed. She was red-faced, preoccupied, and intolerant, much more than before, and finding it difficult to cope. Her contractions were certainly regular, coming one in every three minutes, but sharp and acute, lasting about only about 20 to 30 seconds on palpation.

Mary requested another vaginal examination – she was beginning to feel beleaguered by the relentlessness of surging pain. She was ready to seek comfort in the warm water that she had written so avidly about in her birth plan. Using water as pain relief was imperative to her and central in her coping strategy. My feelings were that she was still in the latent phase, but I knew that for her to hear that would be demoralising. She had coped well so far, and I didn't want her to lose heart. I suggested a cup of tea and some toast as an energy boost and to also allow more time for the contractions to gain momentum. I didn't want to withhold the option of the pool from her any longer than was absolutely necessary (Garland, 2011a, b), but I also didn't want for her to feel beaten if the findings of another vaginal examination were not what she wanted them to be.

Mary declined the refreshments and urged me to perform the examination. She was desperate to know if she had progressed enough to be able to get into the water. I agreed to do this, as it was not contraindicated, but at the same time, I felt slightly anxious that her cervical dilatation might not have changed dramatically.

I found her cervix to be soft, 2 cm dilated and 0.5 cm thick. The baby's head was lower (at −1 to the ischial spines) and in a left occipital transverse position (Sweet, 1997). Although there was progress, Mary was still not in 'established labour'. Indeed, descent and rotation had taken place – thus the baby was moving into a more optimal position for labour (Stables, 2001a), but I knew Mary would only want to hear she had at least reached the magic '4 cm' dilatation. She was becoming impatient and intolerant of enduring painful contractions, without the compensation of speedier progress. I hoped to placate her by telling her in an optimistic way that these were subtle, positive changes. Mary was tired and disheartened; so, it was important for me to help her understand that the cervical and positional changes that had taken place so far were significant, and that a long latent phase is normal (RCM, 2012a).

Mary listened, and though she understood what I was saying to her, it didn't change her overwhelming 'longing' to get in the water, as she pleaded with me saying 'I just need to use the pool; I know I can do it if I get in the pool'. At this point, she became desperate and started to panic. I tried to console her, but verbal reassurance was not enough, she was relying on the water as her salvation. I knew that getting in the pool would bring Mary some much-needed respite, some comfort, some breathing space. I considered the water to be a positive intercession in Mary's prolonged latent phase.

Why make her wait any longer? I decided the time was right, the pool was run and in she got!

The moment Mary entered the water her entire body language and facial expression changed – it was overwhelming to see such a dramatic difference in her demeanour. The tension literally left her body. She smiled and dropped her shoulders as she immersed herself under the soothing, gently warm water (NICE, 2014). I had never seen the pool have such a profoundly beneficial effect on anyone before. I wondered if her contractions would space due to the potency of the analgesic effects of the water (Baston & Hall, 2009) and I decided at this point, it didn't matter. Mary had been resolute, determined in her belief that the pool would help her cope and from the very first instance, it did. Mary's contractions did not space, they continued to become powerful and effectual – her body evolved into a state of uninhibited authority in this labour and I was thrilled for her. At that moment, I realised the importance of considering not only a woman's physical requirements, but also her emotional and psychological needs in relation to pain relief (NICE, 2014).

By the time of her next vaginal examination four hours later, Mary had established in her labour. She continued to make excellent progress following this and she had a beautiful waterbirth in the early hours of the following morning. The pool continued to be the answer for her. It seemed to quietly assist Mary through her whole labour journey: from providing respite during a prolonged latent phase, to ultimately helping to facilitate a natural, unassisted birth.

Mary used the power of the water to meet her physical and psychological needs. She innately believed that the water would help her reach established labour and to achieve a normal birth … and she was right!

Turning anger into serenity: Catriona Cusick

I was caring for a labouring woman who was supported by her partner and mother. I could see that Bea was extremely angry and tired; she seemed so exhausted that she didn't even want to talk. As I helped her to a room, I could see that Bea's body language was guarded. She was not coping well, and she appeared to be so cross, even unhappy. She shouted at me, saying that she had been contracting painfully for the last 20 hours. She was experiencing a long latent phase. Her anguish was utterly understandable, but her attitude was clouding her ability to cope. When she did speak, it was bordering on the abusive. Bea's partner was also becoming upset. Her anger and anxiety were mainly directed at her partner and mother, but also occasionally at me. The atmosphere in the room was rather tense. I was thinking 'I will need to be creative to overcome this anger and negative attitude'. Thoughts of the water came to mind.

After spending a couple of minutes talking to Bea, she started to become more relaxed. I asked her if I could palpate her abdomen. She lay on the bed and with her consent (NICE, 2017b); I commenced the palpation, whilst also assessing the nature of her contractions. They were moderate in strength and lasting approximately 30 seconds and irregular in frequency.

After this, I felt that she was calm enough for me to listen to her baby's heart rate. I used the Pinnard stethoscope, a tool that I find useful to determine and confirm my diagnosis of the position of the baby (Wickham, 2002); then I used a sonic aid as a way of helping this unhappy couple to feel relaxed and reassured on hearing their baby's heart rate. I explained the details of the assessment to Bea and her partner.

Based on my experience, I thought it was likely that Bea was in the latent phase of labour (NICE, 2017c). She became more distressed and really upset at hearing this and said, 'I can't do it, I can't do it, I can't do it' and started to panic. I reassured her and talked her through the contractions whilst gently stroking her arms; she became calmer and at the same time, I felt we started to connect.

We discussed options and my advice was for Bea to return home where she would hopefully feel more at ease and would be able to take a bath, something she had mentioned in her birth plan. However, Bea did not want to go, she felt that being at home would not help her. One reason she gave was the 'dreadful' car journey, because she felt unable to move into a comfortable position; this was something, she said, she could not face again. We continued our conversation and I could feel that Bea and I were now building a rapport. I didn't want us to lose the connection. So, I asked Bea what she would like to do and second, how I could help her.

Bea wanted to have an assessment to ascertain the dilation of the cervix. I explained the nature of dilatation and the changes that occur in the cervix during the latent phase (Mitchell et al., 1977). I also explained that a vaginal examination is not the only tool used to determine the stage of labour (Enkin et al., 2000) but I totally understood Bea's wishes, as knowing the extent of her cervical dilatation would provide her with a starting point and as humans we often like to plan (Walsh, 2000).

I completed the procedure and relayed my findings to Bea and her partner. The examination confirmed what I had expected. Bea's cervix was 2 cm dilated, 2 cm long, soft in consistency, and in a posterior position. The baby's head was −2 to the ischial spines and I could also feel the membranes were intact. Bea was visibly upset about the findings so I asked her again how she felt I could help and support her. Bea repeatedly shouted that she did not want to go home. Her anger and aggression were once again palpable. She was being particularly rude to her partner and I found it difficult trying to calm her during her next contraction.

I left the couple to give them space and went to discuss the findings with my colleague. I thought about suggesting the birthing pool to Bea, as she might find it comforting. I was also thinking about her contractions and how the water would affect her labour (Eriksson et al., 1997). I agree with the notion that relaxation may allow the body to release endorphins, reduce anxiety, and the effect of stimulating adrenaline allows labour to progress naturally (Cluett & Burns, 2009). Consequently, I was confident that the water would help her to progress into established labour.

I took my suggestions back to Bea. I noticed the instant relief on her face when she said that she loved the idea of getting in the pool. I accompanied the couple to the birthing room and helped Bea and her partner to settle in. I was also hoping that this would help Bea and her partner to re-establish their connection too.

I closed the curtains and dimmed the lights to create a cosy environment. Once in the water, I noticed Bea's behaviour was changing, she was no longer angry, irritated, or fractious, and her partner also appeared more relaxed. Now Bea was moving with ease and was able to find comfortable positions in the pool. Bea gave me her first smile and asked for a cup of tea with sugar! She was quiet, no longer guarded, her face changed, and it was truly beautiful to witness these changes in her. The atmosphere was calm and tranquil, and during the contractions, Bea took guidance from me. She was now concentrating on her breathing all the way in and all the way out. Soon Bea's partner took over from me; he had found his 'job'.

I was truly amazed to see the transformation in Bea. By facilitating her needs, she changed from a frightened angry woman to a woman who was now coping with the natural progression of her labour. The buoyancy of water gave Bea the freedom to position herself where she wanted to be. It also gave her the ability to let go of her anger and aggression. The contractions now certainly looked more powerful, but she coped well with them. Bea was very focused and was working hard on her breathing to keep herself centred.

After a couple of hours in the pool, I could see that she was in established labour as her contractions were longer and stronger. I truly feel the use of the water not only gave Bea the space to establish into labour but gave her a means to be comfortable enough and enabling her to find a safe and secure space. I gave her lots of positive reinforcements, which enabled her to trust and believe in herself that she could do it.

I handed over the care to the night shift midwife, said my goodbyes to Bea and her partner and wished them all the best. During the handover the next morning, I discovered that Bea had experienced a wonderful, uncomplicated waterbirth hours later. I was absolutely delighted for them both.

The latent phase and individualised care: Pat Hutson

Jane arrived at 07.25 for the second time in 24 hours. I was the midwife that had assessed her the first time, the day before. I had the impression that she was in the latent phase of labour and I had sent her home, with a detailed plan of when to return to the hospital. As soon as saw her, I immediately understood that she was visibly tired and fed up, not very impressed to see me again! Her contractions were still irregular and mild on palpation. She was 41 weeks pregnant with her first baby.

In her birth plan, Jane was hoping to birth on a midwifery-led unit (NICE, 2017d). She had requested that monitoring should be kept to a minimum and she was hoping to use minimal analgesia, not have an epidural, and have as little intervention as possible. However, she also documented that she appreciated that as this was her first labour, she was unsure of how she would cope with the contractions; consequently, she would be guided by the midwives caring for her. She had attended antenatal classes as well as pregnancy yoga, which had included some relaxation techniques that she was hoping to use.

I carried out a full antenatal assessment (NICE, 2018) and explained to Jane that it was not clinically necessary for me to perform a vaginal examination as I felt she was still in the latent phase of her labour (NICE, 2017c). Whilst understanding the rationale behind my advice, Jane requested the examination anyway, to find out if she had made any progress, as she felt this would help her to prepare, mentally, for the rest of her labour. I proceed to examine her in accordance with her wishes. My suspicions were confirmed. Jane's cervix was approximately 1 cm long, firm in consistency, 1 cm dilated, and the presenting part was at −2 to the ischial spines. Unfortunately, Jane was not yet in established labour (NICE, 2017c). We talked about how the research has shown that women who remain at home during the latent phase of labour, have a better and more satisfying outcome of labour and birth (NICE, 2017c). We talked about how staying in her own relaxing, environment was beneficial for her (NICE, 2018). I mentioned how being in an unfamiliar and strange environment, such as a hospital setting, can result in the body's oxytocin production being lessened. I suggested the possibility of going home to increase her chances of establishing in labour naturally.

When I relayed this suggestion to Jane, she became extremely upset and stated that she couldn't go back home. She felt she needed 'something' to help her cope with contractions. It became obvious that Jane needed my support, and I, therefore, took some time to discuss further options with her. We discussed the possibility of going out for a walk and having something to eat in the hospital grounds. Another option would be that she could be admitted to the antenatal ward, with the option of having analgesia (NICE, 2018). However, my impression was that Jane wanted to stay on the unit and use the pool even though she was not in established labour at this point (NICE, 2018).

After discussing the options, Jane remained disinclined to go home and felt she would relax more and become more confident by staying on the unit for a while longer. But she was reluctant to have pharmaceutical analgesia. Jane decided to go out for a walk and have some breakfast. After only 40 minutes, she came back in tears, reporting she 'couldn't cope any more'.

We discussed her options again, and Jane requested to use the pool. Fortunately, I was able to facilitate this request. Jane appeared to instantly relax at this possibility. Whilst waiting for the pool to fill, I offered Jane and her partner some water, tea, and toast, which they readily accepted, as they hadn't eaten for some hours (NICE, 2018).

When Jane entered the pool, she immediately relaxed and became calmer. She was being well supported by her partner who was providing her with sips of water and jelly babies!

Three hours later, Jane stated she would like to try walking around the room. Jane had mainly knelt in the water as this was the most comfortable position and allowed her abdomen to be totally immersed in the water. However, she felt that she wanted to stretch out her legs and get off her knees for a while. Jane got out of the pool and spent the next hour and a half mobilising and using the breathing techniques she had learnt at her yoga classes. The contractions began to get stronger, so she decided to return to the pool for the relaxation the water immersion had, and could, provide. As I hadn't examined her in almost six hours, Jane needed a plan. I suggested a vaginal examination to ascertain whether labour had progressed (NICE, 2018). There had indeed been progress. The cervix was now central, fully effaced, soft and 3 cm dilated; bulging intact membranes could be felt, and the presenting part had descended to −1 to the ischial spines. The fetal heart rate remained at the baseline of 140 beats per minute and fetal movements were both seen and heard during auscultation. These were promising findings. I now thought Jane was establishing in labour and the pool was helping her. I discussed my findings with Jane and she was delighted! My observations from this point were carried out again in accordance with guidelines for established labour (NICE, 2018).

Once back into the pool, Jane became much less interactive with her partner and me. It was clear that she was working hard, using the relaxation techniques that she had learnt. After a further 45 minutes, she requested to use Entonox. I provided this and gave her the instructions on how to use it most effectively (NICE, 2017b). Jane felt this helped her enormously and I felt it had been requested and introduced at the optimal point in labour. The pool, this time, had helped this young woman in her transition from latent phase to established labour.

Jane continued to progress well, resulting in a waterbirth eight hours later. She birthed a healthy 3095 g baby boy. She was delighted with the outcome and reported that the whole of her labour had been an extremely positive experience

The latent phase of labour and fear: Maria Paz Miranda

Eve had phoned us twice in the last 12 hours requesting advice, as she had been feeling irregular contractions for more than 24 hours. She was 41 weeks and a few days pregnant and this, her second pregnancy, was considered low risk.

Eve was concerned about her progress in labour. When she first phoned, her primary focus was to discuss the memory of her previous birth. She was haunted by her first experience and could not forget that she had endured long hours in an antenatal ward. She never went into spontaneous established labour and ended up needing an induction of her labour for prolonged latent phase and rotational forceps. I reflected on the fact that she might have not established in her previous labour because of the unfamiliar environment that she found herself in (Steele, 1995) This time, Eve wanted to stay at home for as long as possible, hoping that her labour would progress more quickly in the relaxed, familiar surroundings. (RCM, 2012a).

On her arrival to the unit, her contractions appeared to be regular and strong, but short lasting on palpation. Regardless of the short contractions, I was expecting her to be in established labour; after all, she was expecting her second child. Her birth plan stated that she would love to have the opportunity to use the pool and to have the waterbirth that she was longing for.

A soon as the couple entered the pool room, her contractions started to space out. They continued to decrease in frequency, until they finally stopped completely. I could see the fear in the couple's eyes. Eve felt and verbalised that what happened to her six years ago was beginning to repeat itself. I tried to make them feel as relaxed as possible and allowed her to communicate her feelings.

I said that I totally understood their frustration and scepticism about Eve's ability to labour naturally. I said that I was prepared to take her feelings seriously and that I would try and help her at the best of my abilities. After a frank and open discussion, Eve was ready to try, to believe that she could do it. We went for a relaxed approach, opting to stay in the room, have something to eat, maybe take a shower, and when ready, mobilise (NICE, 2017c).

We discussed the advantage of setting short-term goals in labour, as anything else feels overwhelming, hence, unmanageable. We agreed that we would wait for one or two hours before checking the contractions, and depending on their frequency and strength, a vaginal examination to assess her progress might be indicated (RCM, 2012b; Downe et al., 2013). To perform such invasive procedure now without the presence of regular contractions was not recommended, (NICE, 2017c), but more than anything, it could have had a very negative impact on her labour.

For the time being, privacy and tranquillity, I thought, was what they needed. I insisted that they should call me if she felt that she required my input. I left them, hoping for the best. My impression was that her labour has arrested as a consequence of bad memories of her previous labour. My plan was to allow her as much time as possible in a low stress environment.

Twenty minutes later they called me back into the room. Eve was crying, saying that she wanted to use the pool, but her contractions were not strong or frequent enough and that she was told by a friend that the water might stop her from contracting, etc.

I reassured her as much as I could. We agreed, to her surprise, to the following plan.

Eve would use the pool for a couple of hours and depending on her contractions, a vaginal examination would be performed to assess her progress and a plan of care would be reformulated between the two of us.

Why? Why not? I was prepared to use the same couple of hours of 'mobilising' in exchange for the same amount of time 'relaxing' in the pool. My plan was to overturn Eve's fear to hopefully enable an increase in her oxytocin levels, which would eventually help her to establish in labour (Cluett & Burns, 2009).

Eve entered the pool and I could see, that instant, how happy she was. I considered that before diagnosis of labour, she had more to gain by relaxing, feeling that I was considering her fears, doubts, and emotional state (NICE, 2017c). Two hours later, Eve was calmer and happier. Her contractions at this point were short lasting and very mild at palpation; but they were back on the scene. Good, I thought. It was time for a re-assessment of her progression. We needed a plan. However, there were other elements to consider.

Being 41 weeks and three days, Eve had an induction of labour date already booked. This fact was a dark cloud in her mind. In the previous two weeks, she had had two stretch and sweeps, hoping that this simple procedure could have started the labour (OUH, 2016). Eve's last stretch and sweep found her cervix to be 2 cm long and 2 cm dilated, in a posterior position, and of a hard consistence – not very positive findings.

However, the findings of the vaginal examination performed by me this time were very unsatisfactory in her view, but positive to me. This time, Eve's cervix was still 2 cm dilated, still 2 cm long, but soft and in a very favourable anterior position. I had a plan. However, I needed to be careful not to provoke any more frustration in Eve. The first option in my plan was to go home to rest and await events. The second option was to stay in our unit, accept a third stretch and sweep and to use the pool if she needed it (NICE, 2017c). Eve cried. She was anticipating the worse, venous cannulation, pain, epidural, and forceps again. I encouraged her to think and focus again on short-term goals.

The couple needed about ten minutes to discuss things privately. I was aware that the clock was ticking. We know that keeping women in early labour in hospital does not help them in the long run (RCM, 2012a). Eve decided to accept the third stretch and sweep. After it, I left the room hoping for the best. I was confident; the procedure was easy to perform, and Eve tolerated it well. The couple verbalised their need to be alone. Eve was hoping that she would establish her labour soon. However, something, I perceived, had changed. She had shifted from a very negative attitude to a more casual and relaxed mood. I felt very excited about it. The labour would establish, her oxytocin level would increase, I was sure. I left them and encouraged them to call me if they needed me.

I looked at the clock. Three hours and 50 minutes had passed since Eve's admission. It was time to intervene and confront the fact that either Eve's labour had arrested or that she was in established labour. Pensively, I went back to the room. I was so happy when I saw Eve in the pool. Now she was contracting strongly and regularly, she was red in the face and working very hard. Her contractions were every four minutes and they were lasting more than 50 seconds on palpation. She was different, almost self-confident I would say. The intrapartum care was commenced. My plan was to give her another two hours before the next examination, unless her contractions decreased again.

After two more hours in the pool and six hours since her admission to the unit, I decided to perform a vaginal examination to assess whether there was any progress. Eve agreed. When she was trying to leave the pool, her membranes broke. Clear liquor was seen on the floor and everywhere. Eve managed to empty her bladder and when sitting in the toilet passing urine, a grunting sound was heard. Trying to be calm and reassuring I hugged her saying that it was probably time to go back to the pool.

Eve then asked for the examination that I had suggested beforehand. In a calm manner, I told her that I would be happy to wait for another hour, as the time frame was still within normal limits. I explained to her that her progress was evident and that it would be better for her to enjoy the benefits of the pool.

I almost did not finish my sentence. Now she was clearly entering the second stage of labour. Her behaviour was chaotic, she started to scream saying that she could not do it and she requested an epidural. A few minutes after this, her beautiful baby girl was born in the pool, fulfilling her desire to have a waterbirth. Active management of her third stage of labour was recommended, as she had been contracting for more than 24 hours (Mavrides et al., 2016). On reflection, I was comforted by the fact that my plan of care helped Eve to achieve the birth she longed for.

Learning points

We hope that our stories have been of interest to you. Helping a woman in the latent phase of labour is always complex; women need all the help that you can give them.

To facilitate and encourage collective discussion and reflection, we have organised the learning outcomes into three themes that we think are relevant to this chapter.

Individualised care

- Every woman and every labour are unique.
- Cervical dilatation is not the only marker of progress in labour.
- Be holistic in your approach when assessing women during the latent phase of labour.
- We need to be able to provide women with good, tailored, and consistent psychological support during the latent phase.

- Be aware of the impact of fear and anxiety in the complex process of establishing in labour.
- It is important to let women know you are 'listening' to them when they voice their concerns.
- Being able to show compassion is essential when caring for someone, especially when they are in pain.

Creativity

- Be flexible in your practice. Adapt your knowledge and skills to meet the needs of the woman.
- Try to get a feel for the situation; 'read the room'; use your intuition and listen to your inner voice and experience.
- Try to allay fear and word your advice in a way that is positive, helpful, and honest.

Professionalism

- Always consult and consider your guidelines.
- Work in partnership with the woman, fostering a relationship that is based on mutual trust and respect.

References

Baston, H. & Hall, J., 2009. Non-pharmacological methods of coping with labour. In: M. McCubbin & S. Black, eds. *Midwifery Essentials Labour*, vol. 3. Edinburgh: Elsevier, p. 45.

Cluett, E. R. & Burns, E., 2009. Immersion in water in labour and birth. *Cochrane Library*. [Online] Available at: http://onlinelibrary.wiley.com/doi/10.1002/14651858. CD010088.pub2/full [Accessed 28 October 2017].

Downe, S., Gyte, G. M. L., Dahlen, H. G., & Singata, M., 2013. Routine vaginal examinations for assessing progress of labour to improve outcomes for women and babies at term. *Cochrane Library*. [Online] Available at: http://onlinelibrary.wiley. com/doi/10.1002/14651858.CD010088.pub2/full [Accessed 28 October 2017].

Enkin, M., Keirse, M., Neilson, J., Crowther, C., Duley, L., Hodnett, E., & Hofmeyr, J., 2000. *A Guide to Effective Care in Childbirth*, 3rd edition. Oxford: Oxford University Press.

Eriksson, M., Mattson, L.-A., & Ladfors, L., 1997. Early or late bath during the first stage of labour: a randomised study of 200 women. *Midwifery*, 13(3), 146–148.

Garland, D., 2011a. Robust clinical care. In: *Revisiting Waterbirth: An Attitude to Care*. Basingstoke: Palgrave Macmillan, p. 83.

Garland, D., 2011b. Why Water? In: *Revisiting Waterbirth: An Attitude to Care*. Basingstoke: Palgrave Macmillan, p. 25.

Mavrides, E., Allard, S., Chandraharan, E., Collins, P., Green, L., Hunt, B. J., Riris, S., & Thomson, A. J., on behalf of the Royal College of Obstetricians and Gynaecologists,

2016. Prevention and management of postpartum haemorrhage. *BJOG*, 124, e106–e149. [Online] Available at: https://obgyn.onlinelibrary.wiley.com/doi/epdf/10.1111/1471-0528.14178 [Accessed 10 October 2017].

Mitchell, M. D., Flint, A. P., Bibby, J., Brunt, J., Arnold, J. M., Anderson, A. B., & Turnbull, A. C., 1977. Rapid increases in plasma prostaglandin concentrations after vaginal examination and amniotomy. *British Medical Journey*, 2, 1183.

NCT, 2018. Tips on encouraging a straightforward birth during labour. [Online] Available at: www.nct.org.uk/birth/encouraging-straightforward-birth-what-do-labour [Accessed 16 February 2018].

NICE, 2014. Pain relief in labour. [Online] Available at: https://pathways.nice.org.uk/pathways/intrapartum-care/pain-relief-in-labour#content=view-node%3Anodes-pain-relieving-strategies [Accessed 16 February 2018].

NICE, 2017a. Intrapartum care for healthy women and babies. NICE Guidelines [CG190] Initial assessment. [Online] Available at: www.nice.org.uk/guidance/cg190/chapter/Recommendations#initial-assessment [Accessed 15 February 2018].

NICE, 2017b. Care in established first stage of labour; Provide supportive care and information. [Online] Available at: https://pathways.nice.org.uk/pathways/intrapartum-care#path=view%3A/pathways/intrapartum-care/care-in-established-first-stage-of-labour.xml&content=view-node%3Anodes-provide-supportive-care-and-information [Accessed 24 March 2018].

NICE, 2017c. Intrapartum care for healthy women and babies. NICE Guidelines [CG190]. Latent first stage of labour. [Online] Available at: https://www.nice.org.uk/guidance/cg190/chapter/Recommendations#latent-first-stage-of-labour [Accessed 12 January 2018].

NICE, 2017d. Intrapartum care for healthy women and babies. NICE Guidelines [CG190]. Place of birth. [Online] Available at: https://www.nice.org.uk/guidance/cg190/chapter/Recommendations#place-of-birth [Accessed 29 January 2018].

NICE, 2018. Care in established first stage of labour. [Online] Available at: https://pathways.nice.org.uk/pathways/intrapartum-care#path=view%3A/pathways/intrapartum-care/care-in-established-first-stage-of-labour.xml&content=view-index [Accessed 29 November 2017].

OUH, 2016. Oxford University Hospitals Foundation Trust. Maternity information leaflets. [Online] Available at: www.ouh.nhs.uk/patient-guide/leaflets/files/13949Pinduction.pdf [Accessed 28 November 2017].

RCM, 2012a. Clinical practice and guidance/evidence-based guidelines-latent phase. [Online] Available at: www.rcm.org.uk/clinical-practice-and-guidance/evidence-based-guidelines [Accessed 15 March 2018].

RCM, 2012b. *Evidence Based Guidelines for Midwifery-Led Care in Labour: Good Practice Points*, 5th edition. London: The Royal College of Midwives Trust.

Stables, D., 2001a. Malposition and cephalic malpresentations. In: *Physiology in Childbearing with Anatomy and Related Biosciences*. Edinburgh: Bailliere Tindall, p. 519.

Stables, D., 2001b. The onset of labour. In: *Physiology in Childbearing with Anatomy and Related Biosciences*. Edinburgh: Bailliere Tindall, p. 444.

Steele, R., 1995. Midwifery care during the first stage of labour. In: J. Alexander, V. Levy, & S. Roch, eds. *Aspects of Midwifery Practice. A Research-Based Approach*, 1st edition. London: Macmillan, pp. 24–47.

Sweet, B., 1997. Malpositions of the fetal head. In: B. Sweet & D. Tiran, eds. *Mayes Midwifery: A Textbook for Midwives*, 12th edition. Edinburgh: Bailliere Tindall, pp. 631–636.

Walsh, D., 2000. Assessing women's progress in labour. *British Journal of Midwifery*, 8(7), 449–457.

Wickham, S., 2002. Pinard wisdom tips and tricks. *Practicing Midwife*, 5(9), 2.

Chapter 3

The first stage of labour and the water

Maria Paz Miranda, Sian Marie Barnard, Catriona Cusick, and Pat Hutson

Introduction

The definition of the first stage of labour:

> [W]here there are regular painful contractions and there is progressive cervical dilatation from 4 cm.

> (NICE, 2017c)

Ascertaining if a woman has reached the first stage of labour is a challenging aspect of our practice. The responsibility is great and it rests firmly on the midwife's shoulders.

Over the years, the definition of the first stage of labour, based on cervical dilatation, has changed. In 1994, The World Health Organisation (WHO, 1994) formulated intrapartum guidelines where the first stage of labour is diagnosed at 3 cm of cervical dilatation (Cassidy, 1999a). Currently, the WHO recommends diagnosis of the active first stage of labour at 5 cm (WHO, 2018). However, The American Congress of Obstetricians and Gynaecologists (ACOG, 2017) proposed that 5–6 cm of cervical dilatation is desired for a woman to be in the first stage of labour, and therefore, to be admitted to a labour ward (Hanley et al.. 2016).

In the UK, under the umbrella of NICE and local trust guidelines, 4 cm of cervical dilatation and regular contractions associated with progressive cervical changes (NICE, 2017c), are considered the triad of conditions that enable us to diagnose the first stage of labour. However, experience illustrates how it is not unusual for a woman to demonstrate first stage of labour behaviour but have a cervical dilatation of only 2–3 cm. In the same line, there are some women where despite being 4 cm or even 5 cm dilated, their contractions are weak and not strong enough to make them progress into the next stage, and their behaviour is the one of women in the latent phase, taking long hours before they reach the first stage of labour of labour.

It is our duty as midwives to be able to spot the signs of the first stage of labour and act accordingly. Early recognition of the phenomena and the provision of appropriate support and trust in a woman's ability to labour spontaneously are essential prerequisites to be able to give women the maximum possibilities to labour naturally and achieve a vaginal birth. We believe that the timely diagnosis of the first stage of labour, coupled with optimal support in a suitable labour environment, will increase the incidence of normal birth, lower the risk of intervention, and ensure superior levels of safety and maternal satisfaction (RCM, 2012a). Furthermore, misdiagnosis, as well as premature and inappropriate admission in the latent phase, is likely to interfere in the natural process of labour as early admission to labour ward is known to be associated with increased levels of obstetric intervention (RCM, 2012c). The negative consequence of this results in women losing control, creating high levels of maternal dissatisfaction.

These stories will give you examples of women who have been admitted to our unit in the first stage of labour and have progressed smoothly, without complication or delay, achieving a normal birth, supported by our powerful ally: the water.

Water opens a channel of communication: Sian Marie Barnard

Vita arrived on the unit in the late afternoon, surrounded by an entourage of very concerned looking extended family. The only clue I had that she was in pain was that every few minutes, she bent her knees, crumpled her body into Krishna, her supportive husband, and her huge, beautiful, brown eyes filled with tears, which she stared at me through until the pain had passed. She appeared to be in the first stage of labour and I instantly thought of the pool to help her continue towards a lovely, natural birth.

Vita was of Sri Lankan origin and though she seemed to understand what I said to her, she spoke very little English. Her husband Krishna was her birthing partner, and from the very beginning of our encounter, he made it very clear to me that he was there to help in any way he could.

As I guided the couple into the admission room to proceed with my usual admission observations (NICE, 2017c), I asked Krishna to explain some of the subtle nuances that I needed Vita to understand for me to perform the assessment with her full consent. I acknowledged the potential for the language barrier between Vita and I leading to the potential for her choices not being heard; however, I felt the need for an interpreter was not necessary. I could see the channel of communication was open and honest based on Vita's reactions towards Krishna. His support seemed essential to her, as she cuddled into him every time she had a contraction and he responded sensitively and appropriately. They were bonded and close. The emotional and physical connection I observed led me to believe the relationship was mutually respectful and healthy. I was confident that Krishna was communicating Vita's wishes in a truthful way (Garland, 2011) and that he was the person she was naturally turning to as her birth partner (WHO, 2018; RCOG, 2016).

Vita was 39 weeks and five days into a low risk, first pregnancy. The foetal heart rate (FHR) was optimal (NICE, 2018) and a good history of foetal movements reported. Vita's contractions were regular, lasting 50 seconds and strong on palpation, with three minutes of respite in between them. As I performed the abdominal palpation, Vita grasped my wrist and held firmly as each contraction ensued, fixing her gaze on me for its duration. I felt that if I could continue to gain Vita's trust and nurture our midwife/mother relationship, in an environment where she would feel clinically and psychologically safe (WHO, 2018), she would ultimately gain the strength and confidence in her ability to cope during labour (Meredith & Hugill, 2017; Garland, 2011).

Vita had been having contractions since the early hours of the morning. Though she was labouring silently, to me, her tears were a sign of the pain she was enduring. I offered to perform a vaginal examination (NICE, 2017e), to which Vita agreed. Her cervix was 5 cm dilated and fully effaced. The membranes were intact, with the baby's head at −2 to the ischial spines, but in a left occipital transverse, asynclytic, and slightly deflexed position (Sweet, 1997). Although her cervical dilatation was positive, I knew that a proactive approach to correct the malposition would be key to Vita continuing the good progress she had already made; she would need to be mobile to encourage the flexion, rotation, and descent of the baby's head (Sweet, 1997). The pool was the ideal solution, as the buoyancy the water provides enables a freedom of movement that can help to resolve this type of malposition (Burns, 2004). I explained both the findings of the vaginal examination, and my rationale for suggesting the pool to Vita and Krishna; they listened, intently.

Although Vita's facial gestures and body language indicated that she understood everything I had said, once again I wanted Krishna to go over the plan of care with her in detail, just to make sure she was happy with it. Finally, I made sure they both understood the importance of Vita complying with getting out of the water immediately if requested to do so, as sometimes, in an emergency, women must (Morrin, 1997).

Vita's eyes met mine. She nodded in agreement as she started to undress herself in preparation for getting in the pool. I wondered if she would feel comfortable with this; perhaps de-robing in front of me would be an issue, but her cultural identity did not seem to influence her behaviour about this aspect. She seemed completely at ease with her body; it was as if nakedness was a very natural state for her. Her non-verbal cues and body language signalled to me that she was perfectly comfortable and relaxed with the situation. We were effectively communicating, both between ourselves and with the help of Krishna when appropriate.

'Ok then', said Krishna, 'Does she get in now?!'

'Absolutely!' I replied.

'Thank you, Marie', Vita said, as she took my hand to steady her on her ascent on to the steps and into the pool.

I was curious as to how Vita would react to being in the water; this was a new concept for both her and Krishna. Perhaps she would get in and not like it at all, and then we would then have to think again. But from the moment she lowered herself down into the water, I observed an instant change in Vita's body language. She dropped her shoulders, gave a long-sustained exhalation breath, and relaxed. Krishna was taken aback by Vita's immediate change in demeanour and delighted in her new-found tranquillity in the pool. She was subtly discovering an inner strength that was sure to have a profoundly beneficial effect on how she would cope with the coming contractions. There were no more tears, not that it would have mattered if there were. Instead, she just closed her eyes and found her centre, focussing on only the contraction, climbing each one with slow, deep breaths in, and long, slow exhalation breaths out. It was as if the water helped Vita initiate a self-taught breathing technique that didn't involve any verbal guidance from me at all. I was absolutely thrilled the pool was having the desired effect!

I was reassured that maternal and foetal observations were completely normal (NICE, 2017a) and I just wanted Vita to revel in her the bliss of the sanctuary that the pool provided. Krishna continued in his quest to unceasingly support Vita from the side of the pool, encouraging, reassuring, and nurturing his wife towards the realisation birth; his devotion to Vita was extremely touching.

After a couple of hours, Vita was feeling very tired, despite her having been kept well hydrated and nourished. At times like this, getting out of the pool and making a trip to the toilet can be a measure that is enough to change the dynamic and reenergise. Not only was its time for Vita to empty her bladder (NICE, 2017a), but the physical act of getting out of the pool requires the woman to mentally regroup and focus on practicalities.

I noticed that whilst out of the water, Vita seemed to find the contractions much more difficult to manage again. She reverted to her previous behaviour, which was holding her breath and resisting the contraction and panicking, rather than breathing through it as she had done in the pool; she seemed much more vulnerable to the intensity of the pain.

She managed to empty her bladder quickly and without delay, got straight back in the pool. Literally, with the very next contraction, I could see the overwhelming difference the water made to Vita's coping strategy. It seemed to enable her to instantly focus on her breathing again and psychologically climb 'with' the contraction rather than struggle 'against' it. She regained her composure and found her inner resolve once again. The water was a very powerful ally for her; it was fascinating to witness such a strong compatibility.

My shift was coming to an end and I was so sad to have to make my parting gestures to Vita and Krishna. But I was also happy that things were looking so positive for her. I could see signs of imminent transition: traces of bloody show in the water, a protruding sacrum, and distended sacral cleft and rectal 'pressure' developing with contractions (Morrin, 1997). I was thrilled that this woman, who didn't even know that water immersion in labour was an option, was now progressing towards the second stage with such fortitude. To my delight, I learnt that only a few hours after I left, Vita gave birth to a beautiful baby girl, born in the pool!

The power of a mother and daughter relationship: Catriona Cusick

Kaye was expecting her first baby and called our midwifery-led unit two days after her baby was due. Whilst on the phone, I could hear her response to the contractions; she felt they were strong and painful, mainly at the front of her abdomen and down her legs (Labor & Maguire, 2008). In between contractions, she managed to tell me that she had taken a warm bath and she was thinking that she would like to labour in the pool. She felt she was in labour and wanted to come to the unit to be assessed (RCM, 2012a). Kaye arrived 30 minutes later accompanied by her mother. Kaye was very open about her personal circumstances; her partner had left her a few months ago and she was going to be a lone parent. I felt for her, but I could see that she and her mum had a special bond; they seemed to share closeness and honesty that I was sure would help Kaye cope with labour.

Kaye was eager to know how she was getting along. I offered to examine her vaginally to ascertain the stage of labour where she was at. Her cervix was 5 cm dilated and thin, very well applied to the baby's head. She was in her first stage of labour and it was time to start intrapartum care as per guidelines (NICE, 2017a).

Kaye got into the water and straight away 'loved' it. The buoyancy of the water was definitively helping her with the heaviness that she was feeling (Cluett & Burns, 2009). She said the freedom of movement was easing the tightening sensations in her thighs. As the contractions became more intense, she would call out to her mum saying, 'it really hurts mum'.

Her mum would stroke her hair saying: 'remember I told you that it would get strong, you are doing the right thing breathing through the contractions, I am so proud of you'. I watched and stepped back as the two of them related to each other with love and kindness. This was their shared experience.

I listened to the baby's heart rate every 15 minutes and completed maternal observations as per guidelines (NICE, 2017a). I reminded Kaye to drink enough fluid to keep hydrated and to empty her bladder regularly. Kaye continued to use the water and adopted various positions. She favoured kneeling with her arms as a resting place for her head between the contractions and squatting and gently bouncing during contractions.

After a couple of hours, I felt Kaye had reached the transitional stage. The contractions were now every two minutes and she had hardly any time to catch her breath; she started to become fearful and was no longer able to rest in between each one. Kaye was worried about how she was going to cope with a new baby and started to cry, 'what's wrong with me, why didn't he want me?!' Kaye's mum was right there, saying: 'it's his loss, not only is he missing out on being with my beautiful, funny daughter but also on the joys of being a father to this baby girl or boy'. Another contraction came, and Kaye said she had had enough of this and wanted to go home. Her mother and I gently smiled at each other in knowing recognition of this feeling.

It was four hours since her last vaginal examination and my plan was to offer Kaye a further assessment (NICE, 2017a), which she accepted. Her cervix was now 8 cm and the membranes were bulging, I really thought they would rupture during the examination, but they didn't. I could feel the baby's posterior fontanelle centrally, which indicated to me that the baby was in a well flexed, occipital anterior position (Sweet, 1997); the vertex was at the ischial spines. I explained this was good progress. Kaye's mum was delighted with this news, but Kaye was disappointed and a bit despondent, wishing she was nearer to the birth. She was feeling a lot of pain. Her mum and I gave her lots of reassurance, saying that she was doing fantastically. Kaye then requested further pain relief; it was too much for her. She wanted to use Entonox, so I suggested for her to get back into the pool whilst I got this ready. As she submerged herself under the warm water, I could see that she appreciated the buoyancy and freedom of movement the pool provided.

Kaye was most definitely progressing towards the second stage of labour and becoming more vocal with each contraction. She was making a low grunting sound, the sound of pushing. She was squatting and using the sides of the pool to support and balance herself. She said she could feel her baby moving down and that the pressure was very strong. She also felt she wanted to go the toilet to empty her bowels. I reassured her, telling her that this sensation was normal.

I could clearly see that Kaye was now involuntarily pushing with every contraction. I didn't feel it was necessary to confirm full dilation by means of another vaginal examination (NICE, 2017b), because I didn't want to interrupt her natural rhythm. She was totally absorbed in the process and I was concerned that if I disturbed this, it may change her focus, so I decided to wait and see. I continued to listen to the baby's heart rate as per guidelines in second stage (RCM, 2012b). I was anticipating the possible rupture of Kaye's membranes, but this didn't happen; they remained intact. Her mum's encouragement and support were extremely touching.

A short period after this, the vertex became visible, phew! My intuition, knowledge, and experience were right; she was in the second stage! Kaye was pushing with every contraction now and she was changing her position instinctively, ultimately returning to her favoured position: kneeling in the pool. I had equipped the birthing room for the birth of Kaye's baby, assembled a resuscitation area, a delivery pack, uterotonic drugs if required, and plenty of towels. Kaye's baby was coming!

She continued to contract every two minutes and as she started to push, I could see signs that her efforts were effective. The water supported her beautifully and I could see the baby's head was advancing. Kaye felt the baby's head as it was being born. I saw the restitution of the head from an anterior position to an oblique, suggesting that the shoulders had adopted an optimal position for birth (Morrin, 1997). The membranes remained intact, so the water was clear. Kaye pushed, and the baby's posterior shoulder was delivered, shortly followed by the rest of the body (Uppal, 2017). It was a treat to witness the rarity of seeing a baby born in the caul ... such a lovely natural birth!

I remembered she wanted to pick her baby up herself and I encouraged her to do so. Kaye's baby then rested gently against her skin. This mother and daughter were delighted to see the new addition to their family. It was emotional for us all. Kaye shared her concerns about being a lone parent and her worries about how she would cope. I reminded her of how strong and capable she had been in labour and that I believed she would become a wonderful mother, able to face the many challenges of parenthood.

The first stage of labour and the gift of life! Pat Hutson

During a busy night shift, I welcomed Charlotte to our unit. She was accompanied by her partner Jason and another couple. Soon after the introductions, I learnt that it was an in vitro fertilisation pregnancy and the second couple were the biological parents of the unborn baby. This was in fact a surrogate pregnancy. This was a new experience for me, to be in the presence of a generous woman that had decided to go through pregnancy and labour to help another couple, who were unable to have children.

It soon became apparent that Charlotte was beginning to establish in labour (NICE, 2017e). Her contractions were coming every four minutes and lasting over 40 seconds, moderate to strong on palpation and she was only just able to speak through them. I decided to take them into a delivery room where Charlotte could start to familiarise herself with her surroundings and prepare for the birth. She had opted for an epidural during her previous labours, and she was adamant she just wanted to use Entonox and water immersion for this, her third labour. She did not want to be offered an epidural under any circumstances. She had researched using the pool and chatted with friends who had spoken positively of their experiences (Nutter et al., 2014; Richmond, 2003). Charlotte wanted to use the pool for labour, but not for birth. She was concerned about the baby's safety under the water. We talked about the diving reflex that babies are born with, which reduces the risk of water inhalation (Harper, 2014; Sekulic, 2014). However, Charlotte still felt that she wanted the pool only for her labour and I was happy to support her in her choice (NMC, 2015). Half an hour after she had arrived she requested to use Entonox, which I provided, explaining how to use it effectively (NICE, 2017d). The pool at this point was being filled in readiness for use. To eliminate the risk of maternal and foetal tachycardia, my plan was to be vigilant with the water temperature as per guidelines (Harper, 2014).

Birth can be a very intimate and personal time and, in most cases, is between a woman and her close birthing partners only. It became apparent very quickly that, although the couples had met up on numerous occasions during the pregnancy, both couples were feeling somewhat embarrassed and uncomfortable by the situation they now found themselves in. I made the room as calming as I could by dimming the lights and putting on quiet, relaxing music. Charlotte, although going through the labour, took charge of the tense situation, and invited the biological parents to prepare for the birth of their baby, by organising cameras, nappies, going home outfits, etc. The couple busied themselves with the task in hand and I could see Charlotte, once again, concentrate on breathing through the contractions, preparing herself for the imminent delivery of another couple's child, who she had nourished and nurtured during the past nine months.

Once the pool was run and the temperature checked, I invited Charlotte to enter the pool when she was ready. Over the next few hours, the atmosphere in the room appeared to be less tense, and both couples began to chat and further acquaint themselves. Gradually, Charlotte began to withdraw from the social, small talk.

She became quieter and more insular, appearing to be concentrating much harder on her breathing. At this point, she asked if she may enter the pool. Again, she stated that she would like to exit the pool for the birth of the baby. Once in the pool, she appeared very wary and unsure of how to position herself and found the buoyancy of the water difficult to manage. Fortunately, her partner suggested getting in with her, to support her so she could 'float' and concentrate on the contractions instead of her positioning. Charlotte readily agreed, and Jason entered the pool. He was holding Charlotte under the arms, allowing her to relax and float securely. This worked beautifully and Charlotte was calm once again. After a further 40 minutes, it became apparent from Charlotte's behaviour that labour was, almost certainly, progressing into second stage (NICE, 2017b). Charlotte began to become very agitated and stated that she was no longer able to go on with the labour. This can be a common reaction during the end of the first stage of labour, as it progresses into the second stage, this being known as the transitional stage of labour. Charlotte then requested an epidural. I suggested she stayed in the pool for the interim period, whilst I organised a transfer to the obstetric unit where she could have an epidural. However, over the next 15 minutes, the contractions appeared to change once again. Charlotte began to sound expulsive and suddenly declared that 'the baby is was coming' and that 'she couldn't do it'. I tried to reassure her as much as I could. I could see her struggling with the pain. However, Charlotte's behaviour changed again. Somehow, she was calmer now that the birth was imminent. As Charlotte's wishes were to deliver the baby on 'dry land', I invited her to vacate the pool. Charlotte declared she didn't care where she gave birth, she just now wanted it over! She immediately apologised. She, obviously, did not want to upset anybody. Very soon after this announcement, I noticed that the perineum had begun to flatten, a sign that the baby's arrival was approaching. Second stage labour care was commenced (NICE, 2017b) and all the necessary preparations for the delivery were completed. During this time, the biological parents, once again, busied themselves with preparations for the forthcoming arrival of their child. They seemed both excited and apprehensive, unsure of their role at this stage. I had never been in this situation before and tried to support both couples to the best of my ability.

As labour progressed, it was apparent that the baby was 'coming'. Charlotte happily remained in the pool, serene and in control of her body and actions. As the vertex became visible, Charlotte invited the biological parents of the baby to observe the descent and birth of their child. The room was quiet and calm but tense with anticipation. The vertex advanced slowly and gracefully under the water. The head was born, with intact membranes, followed, quickly, by the body. Charlotte calmly and quietly picked up the baby she had just given birth to and held him out for his biological parents to see. The baby blinked and looked at them as if trying to familiarise himself with his new mother and father. The atmosphere in the room was electric, not through tension, but with the emotions of both couples – and me. After a short two minutes, Charlotte asked if the umbilical cord could be clamped and cut. She offered this task to the biological father and the baby was passed to its biological mother whose eyes were glistening with unshed tears. I had just witnessed the giving of, surely, the most precious gift ever!

After the emotions had calmed, Charlotte proclaimed that this had been by far the easiest and calmest birth she had experienced, and wished she had considered trying the pool during her previous labours with her own children's births. She was also pleased that she had remained in the pool for the birth as she felt that by leaving the pool at this stage, the ambience in the room would have been altered, and not for the better.

Advocacy, a midwife's privilege: Maria Paz Miranda

Indu arrived at our unit determined to have the waterbirth that she wanted. Her membranes had broken in the early hours of that morning. Clear amniotic fluid on her pyjamas and bed woke her up, making her feel uncomfortable but happy. Having a baby and experiencing a waterbirth was something that she had always wanted since she had finished her degree.

Her antenatal care was mostly carried out abroad where, as part of the initial assessment, she had been tested for group B streptococcus (Corner, 2015) and the result was positive. She had been strongly advised to attend the maternity unit shortly after her membranes broke as the maternal condition is a known risk for neonatal infection (NICE, 2012b). The recommendation was to have her labour induced as soon as possible and the administration of intravenous antibiotics at intervals of four hours until the birth (NICE, 2012a–c; Hughes et al., 2017; OUH, 2016).

When I saw her at arrival, I had no doubt about her spontaneous rupture of membranes (SROM). Her trousers were wet and abundant clear liquor was seen on her pad. She impressed me for her warmness. In a concise way, she updated me about her pregnancy's details. Indu gave me the impression that she was a confident woman, not afraid of what was happening to her.

Indu communicated her plan to me.

Her impression was that her labour was establishing. She needed more time and she was asking me to be her advocate (RCM, 2012c). She did not want, what she called 'any unnecessary intervention'. Although she was happy to stay in hospital and to start the antibiotics, she declined an induction of labour (Greenwood, 2014). She knew that the plan had to be discussed with the doctor on duty that day. Her attitude was positive, and she was happy to engage in a friendly and open discussion about her decisions. However, she was firm about not being induced without having the chance to establish her labour naturally. She verbalised that she had researched the subject and she felt fully aware of the risks and was prepared to be expectant for the next 24 hours. Regular assessment of maternal and foetal wellbeing was part of her plan and she was even happy to be induced after that probation time. Also, she was prepared to consent to medical intervention in the presence of signs of infection at any time.

This discussion took more than one hour. The Obstetric Unit coordinator, the doctor on duty, and my colleagues were all informed. The intravenous antibiotics were prescribed and administrated without any delay, with Indu's consent. My impression was that she was still in early labour, as she had said before. A vaginal examination at that point was not recommended. The doctor offered to discuss her plan again, but Indu gently declined, requesting to be allowed to mobilise within the hospital's grounds instead. We did not see any problem with her request.

I advised her to check her pad regularly and not be gone for more than one hour at a time, so we could check her signs of wellbeing, listen to the foetal heart rate, and reformulate the plan if we needed to do so. For Indu, this plan was ideal.

I remember being worried. Worried about the devastating effect of a potential neonatal infection. Still, she also knew. On the other hand, it is known that not every baby born from a mother tested positive for group B streptococcus will develop an infection (Hughes et al., 2017). However, the potential risk was enough to make me feel uneasy.

After an hour, she returned to our unit. She told me that her contractions were close together, but still irregular in length and strength, lasting only 20 to 30 seconds.

'How are you? How are you coping?'

'How often do you think you are contracting?'

'Can you feel your baby's movements?'

'Have you had the chance to check your pad?' I asked.

'I am ok. I am coping, but I think that I am not ready yet' she answered.

She passed urine and told me that the pad was soaked in clear amniotic fluid. I asked to see the pad myself and Indu was happy to show it to me. Everything was fine.

'See you in one hour' she said before leaving the unit for the second time since her arrival. However, 40 minutes later, she came back. The contractions were long and strong, she was sweating, still in control but clearly different from a couple of hours ago.

'How can I help you?'

'Have you eaten?'

She said that she had tea.

'Can you examine me?' she asked.

We discussed the implications and risks of a vaginal examination. 'With a diagnosis of group B streptococcus positive and spontaneous rupture of membranes, vaginal examinations should be restricted, to reduce the risk of infection' I replied.

'But I need to know where I am in this labour', she said, 'because I believe this is labour now; so, I need you to examine me, and as two hours had passed since I had the antibiotics, I think it is safe to be vaginally examined, please do it', she added.

'If you are OK with it, I need to discuss it with my colleagues, give me two minutes' I said.

I discussed the request with the doctor on duty. She asked me whether I thought Indu was in the first stage of labour. My answer was 'Yes, I strongly believe that she is'.

'Ok do it, but you need to emphasise, in the strongest possible terms, the indication of immediate induction of labour if the findings are not favourable' she replied.

Indu's cervix was fully effaced, anterior, soft, 2 cm dilated and −2 to the ischial spines, the presenting part was very well applied to an anterior cervix. I called the doctor again to discuss the findings.

'I think Indu is in first stage of labour, she will be using the pool and I would follow the protocol for group B streptococcus positive and labour' (Hughes et al., 2017), was my answer to Indu and the doctor on duty. The medical team agreed not to intervene for the time being and let nature take its course, but strongly advised me to examine her vaginally four hours later. The labour should be actively managed (Cassidy, 1999b) they said, and Indu should be transferred to the consultant-led unit if no progress was made in the next four hours. Indu was relieved with the plan. Within the next 30 minutes, she was in the pool, working hard but confident and happy. Five hours later, she felt the urges to push.

We discussed the significance of the rectal pressure that she was feeling. It could be early urges to push, meaning that she had not reached full dilatation yet, or that she was in second stage hence the pressure, the urges. I decided not to perform a vaginal examination for the time being, based on my close observation of her behaviour and physical signs that she was displaying. She couldn't be more in agreement. Indu was red, hot, working hard physically; a purpura line was ascending between her buttocks, thick, mucosy, and bloody show was seen floating in the pool, a flat perineum and intermittent anal dilatation were observed – all reassuring signs (Downe et al., 2013).

The plan was to wait until the urges to push were unbearable. This plan required a great deal of strength and drive. It was not easy, as Indu declined any other forms of pain relief apart from the warm water. She should be able to manage these urges by breathing only. I could see her struggling with the contractions but still very controlled and smiling in between. What an astounding display of human determination! She was truly amazing!

Eight hours since her arrival to our unit and 14 hours after her membranes broke, Indu had her beautiful girl in the pool as she wanted, and 24 hours later, Indu and her daughter were going home … happy.

Indu gave me a big bunch of flowers. I felt lucky to have had the opportunity to have been there when she needed me, by her side, supporting her choice of labour and birth.

Learning points

These four stories about the first stage of labour emphasise the benefits of using water in labour and birth. We would like to share with you some ideas to help with reflection.

Individualised care

- Women have a voice and choice in the planning of their care during labour.
- Midwives must act as advocates for women to ensure women's language and communication needs are met.

Compassion and emotional support

- The role of a birth companion that can openly and honestly communicate the mother's wishes can be invaluable.
- Respect the relationship between a woman and her birth partner.
- Recognise the importance of family and other supporters in a woman's childbirth experience.
- Explicit support, appropriate physical reassurance, and guidance are essential in helping women to cope during a challenging transitional phase of labour.

Professionalism

- Always consider the need for an interpreter when English is not the woman's first language.
- Familiarise yourself with local and national guidelines on waterbirth.
- A sound clinical knowledge base is an essential prerequisite when caring for women using water during labour and birth.

Creativity

- The first stage of labour is not only about cervical dilatation. Contraction characteristics and the woman's ability to cope are useful in your approach when assessing the first stage of labour.
- Aim to be flexible and open minded without compromising on safety.
- Listen to your inner voice and experience.
- Recognise the 'power of the pool' in transition. Warm water can help to calm and reassure women when entering the second stage of labour.

References

ACOG, 2017. The American Congress of Obstetricians and Gynaecologists. [Online] Available at: www.acog.org/-/media/Committee-Opinions/Committee-on-Obstetric-Practice/co687.pdf?dmc=1&ts=20180226T1202586680 [Accessed 30 November 2017].

Burns, E., 2004. Water: what are we afraid of? *The Practising Midwife*, 7(10), 17.

Cassidy, P., 1999a. Management of the first stage of labour. In: R. Bennet & L. Brown, eds. *Myles' Midwifery: A Textbook for Midwives*, 13th edition. Edinburgh: Churchill Livingstone, pp. 424–425.

Cassidy, P., 1999b. The first stage of labour: physiology and early care. In: R. Bennet & L. Brown, eds. *Myles' Midwifery: A Textbook for Midwives*, 13th edition. Edinburgh: Churchill Livingstone, p. 408.

Cluett, E. R. & Burns, E., 2009. Immersion in water in labour and birth. *Cochrane Database of Systematic Reviews*. [Online] Available at: www.cochranelibrary.com/cdsr/doi/10.1002/14651858.CD000111.pub4/epdf/full [Accessed 12 December 2018].

Corner, V., 2015. Oxford University Hospitals, NHS Trust. [Online] Available at: www.ouh.nhs.uk/patient-guide/leaflets/files/12492Pstreptococcus.pdf [Accessed 13 October 2017].

Downe, S., Gyte G. M. L., Dahlen H. G., & Singata M., 2013. Routine vaginal examinations for assessing progress of labour to improve outcomes for women and babies at term. *Cochrane Database of Systematic Reviews*. [Online] Available at: http://onlinelibrary. wiley.com/doi/10.1002/14651858.CD010088.pub2/epdf [Accessed 21 November 2017].

Garland, D., 2011. *Revisiting Waterbirth: An Attitude to Care*. Hampshire: Palgrave Macmillan.

Greenwood, C., 2014. Oxford University Hospitals NHS Trust. [Online] Available at: www.ouh.nhs.uk/patient-guide/leaflets/files/11290Pwaters.pdf [Accessed 28 November 2017].

Hanley, G. E., Munro, S., Greyson, D., Gross, M. M., Hundley, V., Spiby, H., & Jansse, P. A., 2016. BMC pregnancy and childbirth. [Online] Available at: https:// bmcpregnancychildbirth.biomedcentral.com/articles/10.1186/s12884-016-0857-4 [Accessed 19 November 2017].

Harper, B., 2014. Birth, bath and beyond: the science and safety of water immersion during labor and birth. *The Journal of Perinatal Education*, 23(3), 124–134.

Hughes, R. G., Brocklehurst, P., Steer, P. J., Heath, P., & Stenson, B. M., on behalf of the Royal College of Obstetricians and Gynaecologists, 2017. Royal College of Obstetricians and Gynaecologists. [Online] Available at: http://onlinelibrary.wiley. com/doi/10.1111/1471-0528.14821/epdf [Accessed 21 November 2017].

Labor, S. & Maguire, S., 2008. The pain of labour. *Reviews in Pain*, 2(2), 15–19. [Online] Available at: www.ncbi.nlm.nih.gov/pmc/articles/PMC4589939/?report=reader [Accessed 16 February 2018].

Meredith, D. & Hugill, K., 2017. Motivations and influences acting on women choosing homebirth: seeking a 'cwtch' birthsetting. *British Journal of Midwifery*, 25(1), 10–14.

Morrin, N. A., 1997. Midwifery care in the second stage of labour. In: B. Sweet & D. Tiran, eds. *Mayes' Midwifery: A Textbook for Midwives*, 12th edition. Edinburgh: Bailliere Tindall, pp. 385–402.

NICE, 2012a. Neonatal infection (early onset): antibiotics for prevention and treatment. NICE Guidelines [CG149] Intrapartum antibiotics. [Online] Available at: www.nice. org.uk/guidance/cg149/chapter/1-Guidance#intrapartum-antibiotics-2 [Accessed 30 November 2017].

NICE, 2012b. Early onset of neonatal infection. [Online] Available at: https://pathways. nice.org.uk/pathways/early-onset-neonatal-infection/recognising-risk-factors-for-infection-during-pregnancy-labour-and-birth#content=view-node%3Anodes-recognising-risk-factors-for-infection-and-clinical-indicators-of-possible-infection&pa [Accessed 30 October 2017].

NICE, 2012c. Induction of labour. [Online] Available at: https://pathways.nice.org.uk/ pathways/induction-of-labour/induction-of-labour-overview#content=view-quality-statement%3Aquality-statements-womens-involvement-in-decisions-about-induction-of-labour [Accessed 25 October 2017].

NICE, 2017a. Intrapartum care for healthy women and babies. NICE Guidelines [CG190]. Record the following observations during the first stage of labour. [Online] Available at: www.nice.org.uk/guidance/cg190/chapter/Recommendations#first-stage-of-labour [Accessed 12 January 2018].

NICE, 2017b. Intrapartum care for healthy women and babies. NICE Guidelines [CG190]. Second stage of labour. [Online] Available at: www.nice.org.uk/guidance/cg190/ chapter/Recommendations#second-stage-of-labour [Accessed 12 January 2018].

NICE, 2017c. Intrapartum care for healthy women and babies. NICE Guidelines [CG190]. Initial assessment. [Online] Available at: https://www.nice.org.uk/guidance/cg190/chapter/Recommendations#initial-assessment [Accessed 12 January 2018].

NICE, 2017d. Intrapartum care for healthy women and babies. NICE Guidelines [CG190]. Pain relieving strategies. [Online] Available at: www.nice.org.uk/guidance/cg190/chapter/Recommendations#pain-relief-in-labour-nonregional [Accessed 19 March 2018].

NICE, 2017e. Intrapartum care for healthy women and babies. NICE Guidelines [CG190]. Latent first stage of labour. [Online] Available at: www.nice.org.uk/guidance/cg190/chapter/Recommendations#latent-first-stage-of-labour [Accessed 12 March 2018].

NICE, 2018. Intrapartum care for healthy women and babies Guidance and guidelines. [Online] Available at: https://www.nice.org.uk/guidance/cg190/chapter/Recommendations#initial-assessment [Accessed 23 January 2018].

NMC, 2015. *The Code, Professional Standards of Practice and Behaviour for Nurses and Midwives.* London: The Nursing and Midwifery Regulator for England, Wales, Scotland and Northern Ireland.

Nutter, E., Shaw-Battista, J., & Marowitz, A., 2014. Waterbirth fundamentals for clinicians. *Journal of Midwifery Women's Health*, 59(3), 350–354.

OUH, 2016. NHS Oxford University Hospitals Foundation Trust. [Online] Available at: www.ouh.nhs.uk/patient-guide/leaflets/files/13949Pinduction.pdf [Accessed 28 November 2017].

RCM, 2012a. *Evidence Based Guidelines for Midwifery-Led Care in Labour: Good Practice Points*, 5th edition. London: The Royal College of Midwives Trust.

RCM, 2012b. Evidence based guidelines for midwifery-led care in labour. *Intermittent Auscultation*, p. 4. [Online] Available at: www.rcm.org.uk/sites/default/files/Intermittent%20Auscultation%20%28IA%29_0.pdf [Accessed 12 January 2018].

RCM, 2012c. Evidence based guidelines for midwifery-led care in labour. Supporting women in labour. [Online] Available at: www.rcm.org.uk/sites/default/files/Supporting%20Women%20in%20Labour_1.pdf [Accessed 28 November 2017].

Richmond, H., 2003. Women's experience of waterbirth. *Practicing Midwife*, 6(3), 26–31.

RCOG, 2016. /www.rcog.org.uk/en/guidelines-research-services/guidelines/standards-for-maternity-care/. [Online] Available at: https://www.nice.org.uk/guidance/cg190/chapter/Recommendations 1.2.4 2007, published 2014 accessed 11.03. care throughout labour [Accessed 11 March 2018].

Sekulic, S., 2014. Effects of underwater birth on the newborn. *Sao Paulo Medical Journal*, 132, 3.

Sweet, B., 1997. Malposition of the fetal head. In: B. Sweet & D. Tiran, eds. *Mayes' Midwifery: A Textbook for Midwives*, 12th edition. Edinburgh: Bailliere Tindall, pp. 631–636.

Uppal, E., 2017. Mechanism of labour – The interaction between the maternal pelvis and fetal skull. *The Practicing Midwife* (Featured Article), 20(3), 8–12.

WHO, 1994. Preventing prolonged labour: a practical guide. [Online] Available at: http://apps.who.int/iris/bitstream/10665/58903/1/WHO_FHE_MSM_93.8.pdf [Accessed 21 November 2017].

WHO, 2018. WHO recommendations, Intrapartum care for a positive childbirth experience. [Online] Available at: http://apps.who.int/iris/bitstream/handle/10665/260178/9789241550215-eng.pdf?sequence=1 [Accessed 10 July 2018].

Chapter 4

Postpartum haemorrhage and the water

Maria Paz Miranda, Sian Marie Barnard, Catriona Cusick, and Pat Hutson

Introduction

> Primary postpartum haemorrhage (PPH) is the most common form of major obstetric haemorrhage. The traditional definition of primary PPH is the loss of 500 ml or more of blood from the genital tract within 24 hours of the birth of a baby. PPH can be minor (500–1000 ml) or major (more than 1000 ml). Major can be further subdivided into moderate (1001–2000 ml) and severe (more than 2000 ml). In women with lower body mass (e.g. less than 60 kg), a lower level of blood loss may be clinically significant.
>
> (RCOG, 2016)

Postpartum haemorrhage (PPH) is one of the most common emergencies encountered by midwives. The well-known predisposing risks factors for PPH and its management have been standardised and is known by the obstetric team (Mavrides et al., 2016). However, the occurrence of PPH keeps on surprising us. In our case, in an environment where midwives working in a midwifery-led unit are the main carers, a fast and efficient response is crucial.

We believe that dealing with an emergency is complicated as a result of the conjunction of three main factors.

- First, we encounter the difficult task of estimating blood loss. It is known that the obstetric team can underestimate blood loss (Mavrides et al., 2016). Visual assessment, weighing, and quantifying with special devices are the methods currently in use to determine blood loss. The visual method has the downside of an underestimation of the loss. Weighing, on the other hand, has the risk of an overestimation of blood loss due to the presence of other bodily fluids such as amniotic liquor and maternal urine.
- Second, assessment of blood loss in water is extremely intricate, and there is little evidence of an objective method of assessment. We strongly believe that if we are in the presence of steady blood loss, where the water is changing colour rapidly, it is time to call for help, a diagnosis of a PPH should be made, and the pool evacuated immediately. Our aim is to stop the haemorrhage as soon as possible.

- Third, the ability of the midwife to react and recognise the phenomena immediately is essential (Hancock et al., 2015). Midwives need to be fully aware of the risk factors and how quickly a normal situation can become a serious emergency. Early detection is the key.

These real-life stories will tell you how we manage a PPH after a waterbirth in the pool with differing degrees of severity. The stories look at how we act as a cohesive team, quickly and successfully.

Precipitate labour and PPH: Sian Marie Barnard

On arrival, Louise was talkative and bright. She was 39 weeks into an uncomplicated second pregnancy and although she had a contraction within the first few minutes of coming through the door, I was impressed by how she simply stopped, focussed, and calmly breathed through it. The intensity of the contraction caused her face to flush and her eyes to water, but she managed to smile at me once it had passed. Louise told me she that her contractions suddenly changed from period-type pains when they left home half an hour previously, to feeling 'pressure' and the sensation of needing to have her bowels open in the car as they pulled up outside. Her husband was looking very flustered at the recent developments and was relieved to have arrived safely at the unit!

Within seconds, another contraction came, long strong and intense, this time taking Louise's breath away. This labour had a hurried, precipitate feel to it; the contractions were rushing along and were sudden to reach their peak. I needed to be prepared for an imminent birth. Whilst I quickly scanned the notes to assess Louise's suitability for labouring on our unit, she began to feel an urge to push, but breathed through it. The pool was run in preparation for her arrival, and as this was Louise's second baby, I wanted it ready. This was ideal as on reading her birth plan, I could see she wanted to use the pool.

After swiftly performing the maternal and foetal observations (NICE, 2017c), I offered to perform a vaginal examination, but Louise understandably declined this. She told me she could feel the baby's head was 'not far away' and 'knew' for herself that the birth was close. I was perfectly happy with her decision, as I too felt she would soon be meeting her baby. I certainly didn't want her to miss the opportunity of using the pool!

Once in the pool, Louise breathed a huge sigh of relief. The water's soothing properties seemed to immediately take the 'edge' off the searing peak of the next contraction.

This was a positive situation, but I couldn't ignore the precipitate nature of this labour. Therefore, I was anticipating the possibility of a heavier postpartum bleed (NICE, 2017i). My plan was to await events and be prepared.

Within only a few minutes of her being in the pool, I began to notice a 'drawing together' of Louise's rib cage during her exhalation breath, she was beginning to naturally bear down with her contractions and I could also see external signs of descent present (Morrin, 1997b). I was conscious of the fact that Louise had only been in established labour for 45 minutes and that it looked like I would soon be seeing vertex. With the next contraction, sure enough, I did! The vertex rapidly advanced to crowning with just one push, so I encouraged Louise to 'breathe' through the contraction. It was vital for her to try to slow down and 'control' the birth of her baby's head (Morrin, 1997b). She managed this beautifully and the baby's head was born in a deliberate, steady course. The baby's body followed before the next contraction had even built, swooshing out into the water, pink and toned. Louise gathered him from under the water herself, euphoric in her achievement, greeting him with absolute joy.

Louise spent the next minute cradling her baby in the warm water. I was tentative when I noticed a small, acute trickle of blood disperse into the water, but at this point, I attributed it to possible placental separation (Morrin, 1997a). This is a time when a trickle of blood can easily become a torrent, so I continued to watch avidly. Blood loss in water can be very difficult to quantify (Garland, 2011), and because of this, I wanted to be ready to intervene swiftly if the loss gained momentum. Though it is never my intention to interrupt the first precious moments a mother has with her baby, I wanted to keep Louise safe by managing this crucial stage with a careful eye and sound professional judgment.

At just over two minutes after the birth, blood began to radiate out across the bottom of the pool. I liken this to when lava cascades down the side of a mountain rapidly covering the ground like a red, viscous blanket. This loss then diffused into the water, causing it to resemble the colour of red wine. I could still just about see to the bottom of the pool but could also see a clot of approximately 100 ml in the water. This had all happened within the space of a minute … my feeling was that we were approaching 400 ml of blood loss and with no accurate means of assessing how much more was to come. I needed to act promptly, so I recommended that Louise should get out of the pool for me to be able to accurately estimate and manage any further bleeding.

At this point, I pressed the emergency buzzer to summon help from my colleagues. In the seconds following, I injected one ampoule of Syntometrine intramuscularly, with consent, into Louise's arm (NICE, 2017g). Unfortunately, we didn't have time to allow for optimal cord pulsation prior to the administering the oxytocic. I clamped and cut the cord swiftly. My colleagues streamed into the room within the next few seconds. One midwife helped with the baby (who reassuringly screamed at the top of its lungs at the inconvenience of it all!) by drying and wrapping him in clean dry towels – then passed him for skin to skin with Louise's husband. One of our maternal support workers was asked to scribe.

A second midwife and I helped Louise to climb up onto the step and out of the pool – more blood trickled onto the floor whilst Louise was transferred across the room. We helped her onto the bed, dried her off, and then covered her in a dry sheet and blanket. Louise was still feeling well and lucid, just a bit shaken. I palpated her uterus – it was very well contracted and above the umbilicus and the cord had lengthened, both indications that placental separation had occurred (Morrin, 1997a). There was no bladder palpable and I noticed that Louise had also passed urine in the pool whilst pushing, so I began to deliver the placenta using control cord traction, knowing the bladder had been recently emptied. Another ooze of fresh red blood seeped onto the incopad, it looked like about 100 ml more. I continued the delivery of the placenta, applying steady, consistent, but not over vigorous tension on the cord (Morrin, 1997a). With appropriate downward traction, the cord lengthened further, and as the placenta was delivering, another 170 ml blood clot came with it. I could also see a tear in the perineum that I knew would need suturing.

At this point, I asked for the incopads to be weighed to calculate the amount of blood lost out of the pool so far and for the placenta to be checked – a third midwife was already on the case – good teamwork. With an approximate 400 ml of blood lost in the pool and a weighed 270 ml on dry land, we were at an estimated 670 ml of blood lost. My second midwife offered to site a cannula, take bloods, and administer one ampoule of Ergometrine intravenously (NICE, 2017f) – she prepared Louise for feeling nauseous or actually being sick as this drug is a strong uterotonic given intravenously in the event of a PPH (Lindsay, 1997; NICE, 2017f). This freed me to check the extent of the tear – I could visualise the apex of a second-degree tear and could also see a labial tear which was oozing on inspection. It needed suturing straight away.

Now I needed to stop and think for a second ... is the bleeding under control? Do we need to transfer for obstetric input? I considered our situation and thought not. Louise was feeling well, her uterus was very well contracted, and the placenta was complete; all the appropriate clinical measures had been actioned (NICE, 2017i; RCOG, 2016). Her observations were normal, and the blood loss, although now a PPH at 670 ml (RCOG, 2016) was controlled. If a woman is symptomatic at this stage, a transfer to an obstetric-led care unit may still be required (NICE, 2017i), but this was not the case here. I felt the tear was repairable on our unit because it bled only with the provocation of touch, not otherwise. I discussed the situation with the coordinator, who was also in agreement that given current circumstances, our unit remained an appropriate setting for Louise's care.

I nominated my wonderful colleague to undertake the suturing. She is a midwife that possesses a level of knowledge and expertise that enabled both swift and effective repair, factors which can greatly impact on the woman's psychological and physical recovery from this type of trauma (Baston & Hall, 2009). Haemostasis and alignment were soon achieved (Coad & Dunstall, 2001), with only a further 120 ml of blood lost from the tear, reaching a total of 790 ml estimated blood loss. The procedure was performed with the kind of skill and dexterity that meant that Louise didn't find it at all traumatic or painful. In fact, she maintained skin to skin with her son throughout and even started to breastfeed him before the suturing was finished!

PPH – 'A faint episode': Catriona Cusick

I had met Audrey the evening before when she came to the unit to be assessed; this was her first baby. She was 40 weeks and five days pregnant and in early labour. Her contractions were in-coordinate with some coupling and, on palpation, I felt the baby was in an occipital posterior position. Audrey asked for a vaginal examination to assess the progress of her labour. I found her cervix to be in a posterior position and 1 cm dilated. I recommended that she went home and had a warm bath and to get some rest as she was in the latent phase of labour (NICE, 2017b). Audrey and her partner Peter were happy with this plan. As they were leaving, I wished them a lovely evening, encouraging them to have some fun, suggesting maybe they could to watch a comedy on TV to help the endorphin release which would act as a natural form of pain relief for her. They were totally on board with everything I had said and seemed keen to try the coping strategies I had discussed with them. We had also really gelled during our time together and I was very much hoping to see them again when they came back in.

Audrey and Peter returned only about four hours later. When they arrived, I could see that Audrey was having a challenging time to keep calm during the contractions, her whole stance became rigid, she went up on her tiptoes, and she tended to hold her breath, repeatedly saying 'Oh my god oh my god'. I gently placed my hands on her shoulders, encouraging her to lower and relax them. I then supported her in following my breaths. I slowed my breathing right down, to demonstrate how to take long, deep inhalation and exhalation breaths. Audrey was soon doing this beautifully.

I asked Audrey if she had any birth preferences, and she said that she hadn't. We had a very impromptu discussion about her choices in labour about pain relief (NICE, 2017d). I suggested the pool as an option, but Audrey wasn't sure whether she wanted to try it or not. Never mind I thought, maybe she will change her mind later, although I was sure the water would help her manage her contractions more easily. I could hear Peter talking to Audrey about trying the pool, adding that if she didn't like it, she could always get out. With this, Audrey suddenly made up her mind that yes, she would like to try the pool and once it was filled, she got in.

Audrey's labour progressed normally, and she fully enjoyed the qualities the water can offer. One aspect of her behaviour was quite unusual though; during her contractions, Audrey would duck her head under the water and just let her body float on the surface as if she was in suspended animation. I was extremely curious as I had never seen anyone do this before, so I asked Audrey to tell me exactly how this helped her. She told me it helped her to block everything out so that she could focus purely on her body. Holding her breath and then letting it out slowly seemed to enable a private inner strength. I was fascinated by this and so impressed that Audrey had found such a unique way for the water to help her cope with the pain of labour.

Audrey stayed in the pool for the whole duration of her labour and ultimately gave birth to a baby girl. It was lovely to watch this child being born into the water. I always appreciate the whole wonder of it all. Audrey was so pleased with herself and Peter was showering her and their new baby with kisses.

I had given 10 IU of oxytocin into Audrey's left deltoid muscle in accordance with her wishes for an actively managed third stage discussed prior to her getting in the pool (NICE, 2017g). After appropriate cord pulsation (Burleigh &

Tizard, 2015), the cord was clamped, and whilst Peter was cutting the cord, I noticed a heavy, brisk blood loss. It was more than I was expecting.

I called for assistance as I knew I would need help to get Audrey out of the pool. I was thinking Audrey was having a PPH and I would need to act fast. I explained to both Audrey and Peter that we needed to get Audrey out of the pool as quickly as possible and onto the bed. The colour of the water was now deep red. It was difficult to accurately estimate blood loss in the pool, but I was thinking that it looked as if at least 600 ml of blood had been lost by this point.

The second midwife Clare came into the room and could see immediately what was happening. She pulled the emergency buzzer and requested urgent assistance. I wrapped a towel around the baby and handed her to Peter. Audrey said she was feeling faint; I could see she looked very pale. Clare had drawn up one ampoule of Ergometrine and was just about to administer it intravenously when Audrey fainted. I was supporting Audrey's head, keeping her afloat, and fortunately at the same moment, more help arrived. The bed was moved to the side of the pool and with the use of the emergency evacuation net we success-fully and smoothly lifted Audrey out of the pool and onto the bed (Pidgeon, 2010). I was so glad that my colleagues and I practice pool evacuation regularly on the unit. Once onto the bed I palpated Audrey's uterus which was 'boggy' so I 'rubbed up' a contraction. This worked well, the uterus soon became well contracted and I was able to subsequently deliver the placenta without compli-cation. Whilst I did this, I asked one colleague to administer facial oxygen to Audrey and for the second midwife Clare to site two large bore cannulas (one in each wrist). I requested for the appropriate bloods to be taken and sent off to the laboratory as urgent specimens and for oxytocin continuous infusion to be commenced to maintain uterine contractibility, as well as fluid replacement as per protocol. The blood loss was now minimal.

Audrey then came too as quickly as she had fainted and took off the oxygen mask! She was completely lucid and spoke with clarity. She remembered feel-ing faint and said that she felt ghastly because her tummy was sore. I calmly explained the reasons for this and reassured her that her blood loss was being well controlled. Clare checked the placenta and membranes and reported that they were complete (Harris, 2011). In the meantime, observations of her respiration, heart rate, temperature, and blood pressure were being taken regularly and docu-mented accordingly. Audrey's pulse and respiration rate were initially slightly raised which demonstrated the effect of the blood lost on her circulatory system. However, once I had sited the indwelling catheter in preparation for transfer to the obstetric-led unit, Audrey's observations were already settling to within normal range. I estimated the total EBL to be 850 ml (made up of approximately 600 ml EBL in the pool and a further 250 ml passed onto the incopads on the bed). I quickly inspected Audrey's perineum to assess for trauma and I noticed an ooz-ing vessel. I packed the wound with a large swab to stop any further bleeding and proceeded to transfer Audrey (with baby now skin to skin with her) to the obstetric-led unit for a medical review and perineal repair.

Once she was comfortable in her bed, I verbally handed over all the measures that had been actioned to the obstetrician. She was satisfied that Audrey was in clinically stable condition and asked if I would commence the perineal repair. I was confident to do this, but I made sure that maternal observations were continued whilst I was suturing. Audrey had sustained a second-degree tear. I clamped the oozing vessel with a small clamp and it immediately stemmed the bleeding. I then completed the suturing with the blood loss soon completely under control. In my mind, I was going through everything, making sure nothing had been missed. I was content in the knowledge that Audrey's PPH had been well managed and as a result, she was feeling safe and well.

Once the suturing was complete, the total estimated blood loss amounted to 1150 ml (made up of 600 ml in the pool and 550 ml of weighed blood loss). Audrey continued to feel well with normal observations. I debriefed with both Audrey and Peter. Following our discussion, they understood everything and wanted me to pass on their thanks to the team for attending and being so quick to react and for our calm professionalism. Audrey was so glad to have given birth in the water, despite the slightly hurried exit out of the pool! When I arrived back on our unit, I passed on this feedback to Clare and the others who were present. We reflected on events at length and talked about what we had learnt. We were all delighted that Audrey and Peter were left with a positive impression of their waterbirth experience, despite the complication of the PPH that followed.

Expect the unexpected: Pat Hutson

Karen had experienced a traumatic birth 15 months previously. Her first labour had been induced, with an epidural that took three attempts to site and then didn't work effectively. She had a difficult forceps birth with an episiotomy that broke down in the postnatal period, causing her great distress and pain. When she arrived at the unit, I could see that she was anxious and frightened. She had seen one of the consultant midwives who had suggested she birthed on the unit, which would hopefully help her to achieve a more positive experience this time (NICE, 2017e).

On arrival, Karen was contracting irregularly, giving me the impression that she was still in early labour. After my assessment (NICE, 2017c), my initial impression was confirmed, Karen was indeed in early labour. In normal circumstances, my recommendation would have been for Karen to go home to establish in her labour; however, given her obstetric background and her anxiety, it was obvious that she would not feel comfortable with this. I tried to keep Karen calm in order to optimise her oxytocin levels and promote smooth progress towards established labour. She appeared to be slightly calmer once the observations had been carried out, but the contractions remained irregular. I felt she did not yet appear to be in established labour (NICE, 2017c). We talked about options open to her and, as I initially anticipated, home was not an option she wished to consider. Karen felt that she needed the security of remaining on the unit and stated she would like to use the pool straight away. This is not my usual practice, but due to Karen's anxiety, I thought that by staying on the unit and relaxing in the pool, Karen would benefit from this individualised, women-centred care (NMC, 2015).

Once the pool was run and the temperature was within the recommended range (Harper, 2014; NICE, 2017d), Karen immersed herself in the comfort of the water, instantly, visibly relaxing. Because of her previous induced labour, she hadn't been able to use the pool. This time around, she was feeling that she was able to have her choice of labour and this feeling made her happy and in control. Once in the pool, the contractions remained irregular, every eight to nine minutes, but this state of things did not last long. However, after around an hour, it was obvious that the contractions were becoming stronger and they were now at intervals of five to six minutes. I felt that she was now in established labour and changed the observation timing according to the guidelines (NICE, 2017a–h). Karen carried on breathing through, relaxed and calm. At this point, she asked if Entonox could be used in combination with the pool (NCT, 2018; RCM, 2012), although she felt she didn't yet need it, she just wanted the reassurance that it was there, in the room, ready for her to use.

Another hour passed, and Karen requested to start using Entonox (NCT 2018). Within the first initial inhalations of the gas, she felt she wouldn't be able to use it as it was making her feel lightheaded and out of control but, with some reassurance, she persevered, and it soon became her new best friend! Karen was now using Entonox effectively and appeared to be progressing well. She had been unsure if she wished to deliver in the pool or just use it for labour. At some point, she left the pool and used the bathroom. During these few minutes out of the warm water, Karen experienced another three or four contractions and reported that they were much harder to manage out of the water and wanted to get back in. Again, once in the pool, Karen relaxed and was visually much calmer than whilst out of the water.

Having been back in the pool for a very short time, Karen began to become restless and appeared to be getting out of control of her breathing. I quietly explained to Karen that I felt she was approaching the second stage and all she was feeling, both physically and emotionally, was perfectly normal during this juncture of labour. Whilst having this conversation and trying to get Karen back into her former calm, controlled state, she had one long hard, expulsive contraction and, looking into the water, I could see the baby's head had been delivered.

I was aware that there was also some blood loss at this point. It was a small amount, but as we waited for the next contraction for the rest of the baby to be born, this became a larger amount. I estimated the total loss around 350 ml. At this point, I summoned help into the room, as I anticipated this may result in a PPH. As the blood loss appeared to be continuing, I requested that Karen should leave the pool immediately, explaining the rationale behind it. As she went to stand up, she had another contraction and the baby was born into the pool. The water was now very red, and I estimated a total of over 500 ml blood loss. It was time to act without any delay. To manage the third stage, I gave an injection of oxytocin, first drug of choice (NICE, 2017g), into Karen's left deltoid. The cord was quickly clamped and cut, the baby given to Dad and Karen left the pool. This had all happened within two minutes of the birth.

Once on the bed, Karen's placenta and membranes were delivered normally, although her lochia remained on the heavy side. The total of blood loss now verging on 800 ml. On palpation, her uterus felt boggy, I therefore pulled the emergency buzzer to summon extra help. Whilst waiting for my colleagues to attend, as Karen had only received oxytocin, I gave Karen an injection of Syntometrine, the second drug of choice (NICE, 2017g).

Once help arrived, I took charge and allocated each member of staff a task. Our maternity support worker was given the task of putting out the emergency call for the obstetric team to attend. A student was asked to scribe, ensuring procedure times were accurately documented. Whilst this was all being organised, the other two midwives who attended to my call began siting cannulas, taking Karen's observations, checking the placenta to ensure it was complete, and inserting a urinary catheter. Once the cannula was sited, blood samples for a full blood count and group and save were collected and sent. As Karen was continuing to trickle lochia, intravenous Ergometrine was administered. At this point, the maternity support worker arrived back into the room stating that the obstetricians were on their way, and she began to weigh the sheets, incopads, etc. to ensure an accurate blood loss could be documented.

On feeling Karen's uterus again, I could feel it was now well contacted and the blood loss had started to subside. At this point, the obstetric team appeared at the door. After a succinct handover, they began requesting cannulas, catheters, blood to be sent, etc. all of which had already been actioned. One of my colleagues had just finished working out blood loss, and the total was in the region of 1350 ml (the amount in the pool was only an estimation). Karen's observations had stayed within normal limits and, at this point, she didn't feel symptomatic of the blood loss. The decision, in agreement with the obstetricians, was made for Karen to remain on the unit, with a low threshold to transfer to the observation area if she became symptomatic or started to bleed again. A blood sample to check her haemoglobin levels was requested after six hours to check that it remained within a normal range.

During this time, Karen's partner had been sat in the corner with the baby, and although every effort to reassure him and let him know what was happening had been made, both he and Karen needed a full debriefing about the sequence of events that had just taken place.

Karen made a good recovery in the postnatal period, her haemoglobin came back at 98 g/dl, she remained asymptomatic, and she was discharged home 48 hours post-birth with a prescription of ferrous sulphate.

PPH? Prepare yourself! Maria Paz Miranda

Ann was expecting her third child when I met her. She had been admitted to the unit in established labour in the early hours of that Sunday. Later that day, she would tell me that she had been contracting for the last two days, irregularly. This single piece of information, a prolonged latent phase, put me on guard for a potential PPH. Ann had delivered her two previous babies in a low risk setting maternity unit and she was hoping to repeat the experience this time.

She had the first part of her antenatal care for this pregnancy abroad. Her notes were divided into two different sets. The first set of antenatal notes were from a French-speaking hospital, and the second set of notes were our own Trust notes. Ann and her wife had bought a new house in the area and they were planning to settle down somewhere in the region.

I remember her being extremely calm, smiling at me when I entered the room, enjoying the pool. She was glowing with the perspective of meeting her little unborn boy. The couple made me feel extremely welcome and I felt that the day ahead would be just fine. Her membranes were still intact.

We engaged in an animated conversation, where was she living before, how the health system was in that country, what the food was like, etc. From looking at her, I thought: 'she is too relaxed for a woman in labour ... Should I be concerned?' When I asked at what time the strong contractions started, she told me, for the second time, that she had been contracting like this for the last two days! I started to speculate whether I was in the presence of woman still in a latent phase of labour (WHO, 2018). I was not sure. She had been examined vaginally two hours before; her cervix was found to be 5 cm dilated and 1 cm long, −2 to the ischial spines. I looked at her antenatal blood results again, just be sure. Her haemoglobin level was 103 g/dl, she was vegetarian, and taking vitamins and liquid iron of some sort.

Some warning signs became evident to me:

1   Anaemia (Hb of 103 g/dl).
2   Prolonged latent phase of labour surely!

Due to these potential risks for PPH (NICE, 2017g), I decided that active management of the third stage of labour should be a part of my plan of care (Mavrides et al., 2016; NICE, 2017g). Ann had a simple and sensible birth plan: she was willing to accept any intervention that we considered appropriate. Therefore, accepting the recommendation of an active management of the third stage was not a problem. We discussed Syntometrine as the chosen drug for this purpose. In advance, we decided that the site of injection would be her left shoulder, as she wanted to remain in the pool for a few minutes after her baby was born.

Throughout the whole morning, Ann was having strong and regular contractions. However, for a multiparous woman, I thought, her labour appeared to be progressing slowly. Her cervix was 5 cm and 1 cm long four hours ago. As per guidelines, I should examine her (NICE, 2017c).

On my vaginal examination, her cervix was found to be 5 cm dilated and 1 cm long again, basically, no changes. Ann was not surprised about the findings as she felt that her contractions were still mild in intensity. We discussed the options and she accepted the fact that moving would help. She went for a walk around and her wife took the opportunity to go out of the unit for some fresh ground coffee.

It did not take long for all of us to see big changes. Forty minutes later she was different; she looked compromised by the strength of the contractions, unlike how I'd seen her before. I called her wife. I felt she should be back sooner rather than later. Two hours later, I remember, Ann looked at me and said 'My baby is coming, I can feel it!'

By her side, I kept assessing and reassuring her until the inevitable happened. She felt the strongest urge to push and her membranes broke; pale, insignificant meconium was seen and then, without warning, the baby was born in one push. I called for help, I needed someone else in the room, an extra pair of hands. The rapid sequence of events did not give me time to call for the second midwife in advance, as we usually do. Our lovely and very experienced maternity support worker, Lou, came to my aid. I felt safe, she is one of those colleagues that is always ahead of things, intelligent, practical, and efficient. What a change I thought! Now a prolonged latent phase transformed itself into a precipitate birth!

Ann reached for her baby at the bottom of the pool. She brought him to her chest and smiled at him, crying!

My eyes were everywhere: checking the baby and his respiratory effort, the colour of the water, etc. Everything was fine. Within the next minute, Syntometrine was given intramuscularly to her left shoulder as we had discussed previously. Peace and tranquillity did not last long. Sudden massive blood loss was seen in the water. The water was getting darker and darker, fast. About 400 ml I thought. I was unable to be exact, as assessing blood loss in the water is very difficult. I looked at Lou, she knew the next move. I made a small gesture and the emergency buzzer was pressed. We needed help. I informed the couple about what was happening, and I warned them of the people that would soon be coming into the room to assist me.

Within the next minute, the whole team was in the room. I knew I had a very good team with me that day. I felt reassured and well supported.

I explained that Ann was losing more blood than we expected, and it was necessary for her to leave the pool quickly. I asked Lou to take care of the baby and wife, whilst I was cutting the umbilical cord without delay. Ann was actively bleeding. In a matter of seconds, no more, everybody knew what to do. I stopped to ask one of my colleagues to document procedures and times, and to delegate other tasks. Everybody was expectant, waiting in anticipation of what was to follow.

Ann was helped to her bed and I proceeded to deliver the placenta by control cord traction. After that, the uterus remained soft and high on palpation. She was still bleeding. I started to massage the uterus, attempting to stimulate a contraction to reduce the blood loss, whilst preparing for the next procedure (NICE, 2017i). The incopads were kept and weighed as we were using them, by our efficient Lou, the MSW, already present in the room with the scale. She reported loud and clear that we were reaching 500 ml of blood loss. This, plus the 400 ml in the pool meant 900 ml already. We needed to be prepared to transfer her to our consultant-led unit as we were heading towards a major obstetric haemorrhage and Ann could have needed additional medical input.

Maternal observations were commenced every five minutes using an electronic device. One of the midwives, who was asked to check the placenta and membranes, came back to report that they were intact and complete.

Now, I needed to site a cannula that had been prepared for insertion for me by another member of the team. I took the specified blood samples and I asked one of the students helping to label and send the samples as soon as possible, and report back to me when it was done. She confirmed she felt able to do this. The subsequent step was to give Ann Ergometrine (NICE, 2017i). My friend had it ready. She showed me the ampoule and confirmed the name, dose, and expiry date by reading it aloud. I administered it slowly, intravenously, trying to minimise the strong nausea associated with this drug (NICE, 2017i). Ann was warned about this. We stopped for a few seconds to assess the situation. What else needed to be done? Was everybody aware of their tasks?

Syntocinon infusion and intravenous fluids were commenced and a Foley catheter was inserted as protocol. Lou told me that the blood loss was over 1000 ml after weighing all the incopads. Ann was wrapped in a couple of blankets, awake, in good condition but shaken. Maternal observations were normal, and I took a moment to explain what was happening, and what was next. I told her that she needed to be transferred as protocol for a PPH. The consultant-led unit was aware that a major obstetric haemorrhage had occurred, that first-line management had been activated, and that Ann was in a stable condition. They were waiting for us.

Ann's resilience and understanding of the need to cooperate during this emergency was outstanding. We talked about what happened and I thanked her for her strength. She helped us to help her. We hugged after the event and I left, relieved that further injury was avoided by prompt intervention.

I was shaken and grateful at the same time for the efficient and calm support that I received from my colleagues.

Learning points

Postpartum haemorrhage can be a frightening event, especially if the woman is in the pool. The emergency becomes easier to manage if midwives have regular drills and practice scenarios as part of a cohesive team. We have summarised our learning points from each story. We hope they are of use to you.

Before the emergency

- Consider the presence of risk factors associated with PPH.
- Do not minimise the impact of blood loss in 'low risk' women, especially low BMI women.
- Once the emergency has been diagnosed call for help. The sooner the better.

During the emergency

- If you are leading the emergency, DELEGATE reasonable and single tasks.
- Address people by their names: 'Louise can you please send these bloods?' Ask them to report back to you when it is done.

- If you are not comfortable with the task that you were given, do not hesitate and ask for help.
- It is important to remember that a PPH may have combined causes.
- Always consider the five Ts:

TONE	Is the uterus well contracted?
TISSUE	Is the placenta complete? Consider retained products as a cause.
THROMBIN	Is the blood clotting? Consider coagulation disorders such as disseminated intravascular coagulation, etc.
TRAUMA	Perineal, labial, vaginal wall, and cervical tears need to be assessed and repaired immediately.
TIMELY INTERVENTION	Helps prevent maternal morbidity. Delegate the care of the baby and family.

After the emergency

- Debrief with the family and staff involved in the event.
- Complete all the relevant proformas and incident reports.
- Complete a retrospective account of events to clarify your thoughts and aid reflection. This will enable possible future improvements in your learning and PPH management.

References

Baston, H. & Hall, J., 2009. Perineal repair. In: *Midwifery Essentials – Labour*. Edinburgh: Churchill Livingston, p. 159.

Burleigh, A. & Tizard, H., 2015. Latest recommendations on timing of clamping the umbilical cord. [Online] Available at: www.rcm.org.uk/news-views-and-analysis/views/latest-recommendations-on-timing-of-clamping-the-umbilical-cord [Accessed 15 July 2018].

Coad, J. & Dunstall, M., 2001. The puerperium. In: *Anatomy and Physiology for Midwives*. London: Mosby, pp. 316–317.

Garland, D., 2011. Robust clinical care. In: *Revisiting Waterbirth an Attitude to Care*, 1st edition. Basingstoke: Palgrave Macmillan, pp. 89–93.

Hancock, A., Weeks, A. D., & Lavender, D. T., 2015. BMC pregnancy and childbirth. [Online] Available at: https://bmcpregnancychildbirth.biomedcentral.com/articles/10.1186/s12884-015-0653-6 [Accessed 14 December 2017].

Harper, B., 2014. Birth, bath and beyond: the science and safety of water immersion during labor and birth. *The Journal of Perinatal Education*, 23(3), 124–134.

Harris, J., 2011. How to … perform an examination of the placenta. [Online] Available at: www.rcm.org.uk/news-views-and-analysis/analysis/how-to%E2%80%A6-perform-an-examination-of-the-placenta [Accessed 15 July 2018].

Lindsay, P., 1997. Complications of the third stage of labour. In: Sweet, B, Tiran, D., eds, *Mayes' Midwifery A Textbook for Midwives*, 12th Edition. Edinburgh Bailliere Tindall, pp. 703–718.

Mavrides, E., Allard, S., Chandraharan, E., Collins, P., Green, L., Hunt, B. J., Riris, S., & Thomson, A. J., on behalf of the Royal College of Obstetricians and Gynaecologists., 2016. Prevention and management of postpartum haemorrhage. *BJOG*, 124, e106–e149. [Online] Available at: https://obgyn.onlinelibrary.wiley.com/doi/epdf/10.1111/1471-0528.14178 [Accessed 17 October 2017].

Morrin, N., 1997a. Midwifery care in the third stage of labour. In: B. Sweet & D. Tiran, eds. Mayes' *Midwifery: A Textbook for Midwives*, 12th edition. Edinburgh: Bailliere Tindall, pp. 403–417.

Morrin, N. A., 1997b. Midwifery care in the second stage of labour. In: B. Sweet & D. Tiran, eds. Mayes' *Midwifery: A Textbook for Midwives*, 12th edition. Edinburgh: Bailliere Tindall, pp. 385–402.

NCT, 2018. Pain relief in labour. [Online] Available at: www.nct.org.uk/birth/pain-relief-during-labour#Water [Accessed 1 August 2018].

NICE, 2017a. Intrapartum care for healthy women and babies. NICE Guidelines [CG190]. First stage of labour. [Online] Available at: www.nice.org.uk/guidance/cg190/chapter/Recommendations#first-stage-of-labour [Accessed 29 November 2017].

NICE, 2017b. Intrapartum care for healthy women and babies. NICE Guidelines [CG190]. Latent first stage of labour. [Online] Available at: www.nice.org.uk/guidance/cg190/chapter/Recommendations#latent-first-stage-of-labour [Accessed 15 July 2018].

NICE, 2017c. Initial assessment of a woman in labour. [Online] Available at: https://pathways.nice.org.uk/pathways/intrapartum-care/initial-assessment-of-a-woman-in-labour#content=view-node%3Anodes-assess-woman-and-unborn-baby [Accessed 29 January 2018].

NICE, 2017d. Intrapartum care for healthy women and babies. NICE Guidelines [CG190]. Pain relieving strategies. [Online] Available at: www.nice.org.uk/guidance/cg190/chapter/Recommendations#pain-relief-in-labour-nonregional [Accessed 19 March 2018].

NICE, 2017e. Intrapartum care for healthy women and babies. NICE Guidelines [CG190]. Place of birth. [Online] Available at: www.nice.org.uk/guidance/cg190/chapter/Recommendations#place-of-birth [Accessed 1 August 2018].

NICE, 2017f. Intrapartum care for healthy women and babies. NICE Guidelines [CG190]. Postpartum haemorrhage. Risk factors. [Online] Available at: www.nice. org.uk/guidance/cg190/chapter/Recommendations#third-stage-of-labour [Accessed 18 March 2018].

NICE, 2017g. Intrapartum care for healthy women and babies. NICE Guidelines [CG190]. Active and physiological management of the third stage. [Online] Available at: www.nice.org.uk/guidance/cg190/chapter/Recommendations#third-stage-of-labour [Accessed 18 March 2018].

NICE, 2017h. Intrapartum care for healthy women and babies. NICE Guidelines [CG190]. Record the following observations during the first stage of labour. [Online] Available at: www.nice.org.uk/; https://www.nice.org.uk/guidance/cg190/chapter/Recommendations#first-stage-of-labour [Accessed 18 March 2018].

NICE, 2017i. Intrapartum care for healthy women and babies. NICE Guidelines [CG190]. Postpartum haemorrhage, management. [Online] Available at: www.nice.org.uk/guidance/cg190/chapter/Recommendations#third-stage-of-labour [Accessed 12 December 2017].

NMC, 2015. *The Code, Professional Standards of Practice and Behaviour for Nurses and Midwives*. London: The Nursing and Midwifery Regulator foe England, Wales, Scotland and Northern Ireland.

Pidgeon, J., 2010. Avoiding troubled waters. [Online] Available at: www.rcm.org.uk/news-views-and-analysis/analysis/avoiding-troubled-waters [Accessed 15 July 2018].

RCM, 2012. Evidence based guidelines for midwifery-led care in labour. [Online] Available at: www.rcm.org.uk/sites/default/files/Immersion%20in%20Water%20%20for%20Labour%20and%20Birth_0.pdf [Accessed 15 March 2018].

RCOG, 2016. https://www.rcog.org.uk/en/guidelines-research-services/guidelines/gtg52/

WHO, 2018. World Health Organisation. Recommendations: intrapartum care for a positive childbirth experience. [Online] Available at: http://apps.who.int/iris/bitstream/10665/260178/1/9789241550215-eng.pdf?ua=1 [Accessed 18 March 2018].

Chapter 5

Shoulder dystocia and the water

Maria Paz Miranda, Sian Marie Barnard, Catriona Cusick, and Pat Hutson

Introduction

> Shoulder dystocia is defined as a vaginal cephalic delivery that requires additional obstetric manoeuvres to deliver the fetus after the head has delivered and gentle traction has failed. An objective diagnosis of a prolongation of head-to-body delivery time of more than 60 seconds has also been proposed, but these data are not routinely collected. Shoulder dystocia occurs when either the anterior, or less commonly the posterior, fetal shoulder impacts on the maternal symphysis, or sacral promontory, respectively.
>
> (RCOG, 2012)

Postpartum haemorrhage (PPH) is one of the most common emergencies encountered by midwives when caring for a woman in labour and shoulder dystocia is one of the most challenging complications. This is especially the case for midwives working on a midwifery-led unit (MLU), where the first minutes after the diagnosis, and before the arrival of the emergency obstetric team, are our sole responsibility.

The management of this obstetric emergency has been summarised in a few relevant points by the Royal College of Obstetricians and Gynaecologists:

- Shoulder dystocia should be managed systematically.
- Immediately after recognition of shoulder dystocia, additional help should be called.
- The problem should be stated clearly as 'this is shoulder dystocia' to the arriving team.
- Fundal pressure should not be used.
- McRoberts' manoeuvre is a simple, rapid and effective intervention and should be performed first.
- Suprapubic pressure should be used to improve the effectiveness of the McRoberts' manoeuvre.
- An episiotomy is not always necessary.

(RCOG, 2012)

When we talk about systematically managed, we are saying that there is an established set of manoeuvres to be performed in a certain order. However, when we are confronted by this emergency in an MLU setting (RCOG, 2012), the characteristics of the women in labour become pivotal regarding the order of the manoeuvres. We strongly believe that the manoeuvres follow a 'common sense' approach in the sense that you perform one or another of the manoeuvres depending on the circumstances, that is, maternal position, degree of mobility of the woman, availability of birth attendants, and degree of expertise, amongst other factors (RCOG, 2012). A woman in the pool, alert and fully mobile, differs totally from a bedbound woman with an epidural, who is unable to move fast enough to try different positions. Most of the time, in our experience, the sole fact of standing and lifting one leg to leave the pool allows the shoulders to rotate internally (Coates, 1995; Shiers, 1999). If this does not work, the woman will be helped to abandon the pool, to walk towards her bed, and possibly adopt an 'all fours' position, as the first line manoeuvre, which is described as an appropriate manoeuvre to be used in a community setting (RCOG, 2012). It is an easy manoeuvre to achieve and takes little time for the woman to adopt it. If this does not work, we move promptly to the McRoberts' position, to suprapubic pressure and internal manoeuvres, as needed (RCOG, 2012).

We hope that you enjoy our stories and feel reassured that you can take away any relevant element from these stories that might help to enhance your practice.

Waterbirth and shoulder dystocia – there's no 'I' in team: Sian Marie Barnard

My involvement in this episode of care was initially as second midwife. My colleague Emily called me to assist her in supporting Rose, who was in the pool in labour with her first baby. Second stage had been confirmed by vaginal examination 25 minutes earlier and Rose was finding the pressure and pain unbearable. She was resisting the advice and guidance being offered to her and was losing control. Emily was concerned. As Rose was no longer able to cooperate, Emily was finding it increasingly difficult to accurately listen in the baby's heart rate, or perform any of the observations she needed to during this stage of labour (NICE, 2018b).

I could hear from the office that Rose had become vocal and sounded extremely distressed, and I was not surprised to hear Emily's buzzer summoning me to assist her. Birth sounded imminent, so I felt my presence as second midwife at this time was wholly appropriate.

Between us, Emily and I soon calmed Rose down. We helped Rose to realise the benefits of the water for the challenging transition she was experiencing; as her contractions surged, we encouraged her to allow the pool to work its enveloping, warming magic. Vertex now visible, the water continued to soothe, easing the intense burning sensation of the perineal skin as it stretched to paper thin to accommodate the crowning head (Morrin, 1997). Things were looking good and I didn't anticipate any problems at this point.

09:43: The baby's head delivered beautifully, one hour and 25 minutes from diagnosis of the second stage. This was comprised of 35 minutes of passive second stage and 50 minutes of active pushing – good progress, I thought. Rose was overcome, and so relieved to have done it, to have pushed her baby's head out herself … 'well done, well done!' we said! I was scribing, so I documented the time of this in the notes.

As I looked down into the water though, I could see the baby 'turtle-necking' as if it was trying to draw its chin back in towards the perineum and I noticed that there was no external restitution of the head (RCOG, 2012). Given these signs, my suspicions began to rise. I was anticipating a possible shoulder dystocia, as was Emily.

Our guidelines state that we wait for the next contraction in order to allow time for further rotation and descent which can deliver the shoulders under the pubic arch and facilitate birth (RCOG, 2012); so, we waited … for what felt like a long two minutes for the next contraction. The urge to push slowly built … then Rose gathered her breath … put her chin on her chest … and gave a long, hard push downwards. The baby's head did not move at all.

My heart began to pound … this was a shoulder dystocia.

09:45: Emily pressed the emergency buzzer and Sarah, our maternity support worker, came in. I informed Sarah that this was a shoulder dystocia and asked her to summon the obstetric and newborn teams immediately. I assisted Rose out of the pool without delay. She was distraught and crying: 'Is my baby okay, is my baby okay?!'

Ed, her partner, looked shell-shocked but tried to help us by steadying Rose as she straddled over the side of the pool with a baby's head between her legs. This was a terrifying situation for them, so the need for us to be clear and concise in our instruction was vital.

09:46: Rose was out of the pool and onto the bed – we dried her off as best we could. We assisted Rose's legs into the McRoberts position whilst at the same time ensuring the back of the bed was lowered so the surface was flat (RCOG, 2012). Sarah was asked to scribe and support Ed. Cheryl (another midwife) supported Rose's legs in the McRoberts' position, whilst calmly explaining what was happening to her. Another midwife also came to help. A team of five were now in the room, working together, supporting one another. A second maternity support worker switched on and checked the Resuscitaire and waited outside to direct the obstetric team to our room on their arrival. The baby still had not delivered … no descent, no restitution.

My heart was racing … adrenaline pumping … but both Emily and I remembered – *do not* apply axial traction – pulling on the baby's head before rotation of the shoulders is potentially very harmful and will only further impede the delivery (Stables, 1999). We were painfully aware that the McRoberts' manoeuvre hadn't worked.

I confirmed the lie of the baby's back with Emily, and applied suprapubic pressure appropriately, in an attempt to both enhance the effects of the McRoberts' manoeuvre and dislodge the baby's shoulder under the pubic arch (RCOG, 2012). This had no effect and we saw no change.

09:47: Emily evaluated the need for an episiotomy (RCOG, 2012) and without delay, proceeded to an internal manoeuvre to deliver the baby's posterior arm. She was unsuccessful ... things were extremely concerning now. The emergency team were still on their way. Emily then tried to rotate the baby using an internal manual rotation of 180°, the aim of which was to dislodge the impacted shoulder (Coates, 1997; Stables, 1999) but the baby remained firmly wedged. I cannot convey how frightening and serious things were at this point. Both Emily and I felt desperately worried that this baby was not delivering – but it was imperative that we remained calm and logical – supporting one another, suggesting the next move in order to try to solve this frightening emergency. We constantly encouraged Rose to breathe through her contractions and not to push; we needed to free the baby's shoulders first (RCOG, 2012).

09:48: Emily and I assisted Rose on to her knees into an all fours position. This change in posture can sometimes be just enough to facilitate a change in the internal dynamics by relieving pressure from the sacrum (RCOG, 2012). In this position, I inserted my hand into the sacral promontory and pushed the anterior shoulder forwards to adduct the shoulders, working from behind the baby's back (Coates, 1997). This manoeuvre can decrease the bisacromial diameter, allowing the shoulders to be freed under the symphysis pubis (Stables, 1999), but this didn't work either. There was no change ... the baby was still undelivered.

Emily and I looked into each other's eyes ... we were starting to feel desperate, but we both knew we needed to keep going with our manoeuvres. We quickly conferred and decided to try McRoberts again. Cheryl agreed with us and assisted Rose's legs into position. Again, I attempted to deliver the posterior arm, just as Emily had tried to do previously. I could feel that the baby had its arm braced behind its back and I tried to reach in further and grasp the wrist but couldn't. I was now afraid that this baby was becoming very compromised, afraid that it did not seem to be delivering despite all our best efforts. But we needed to persevere – bolstering one another – repeating our manoeuvres until this baby was free. Rose continued to breathe hard and deep on Entonox managing to bear all of this ... managing not to push with her contractions, which was vital. She was remarkable.

The systematic approach we were using had so far been unsuccessful, but we knew we needed to remain calm and keep going until the obstetric team arrived. Once again, I applied pressure against the posterior aspect of the anterior shoulder (Stables, 1999) and felt some movement. I continued this for a few more seconds then proceeded to apply routine downward traction under the baby's armpit. I felt some more movement, more descent ... thank goodness!

09:49: The obstetric team arrived. Annabel (an obstetrician) observed what I was doing and could see both Emily and I were exhausted and offered to take over. Annabel continued the downward traction I had initiated but felt that the shoulder was not descending any further and so again attempted to free the posterior arm.

Annabel advanced her hand deeply into the birth canal, further than Emily and I had done before. She finally managed to grasp the baby's wrist and pull it forwards, sweeping the arm over the baby's chest.

09:50: The arm was then delivered, and the posterior shoulder was free!

With the next contraction, Emily and I encouraged Rose to push once more and to our great relief, the baby was delivered at 09:51.

I administered one ampoule of Syntometrine intramuscular immediately after birth, in anticipation of a heavy blood loss which could well have followed such a prolonged and traumatic second stage (RCOG, 2012).

The baby boy was initially shocked, not surprising given the eight-minute delay between the birth of his head and his body and the manoeuvres he had endured. But I could see straight away that he had tolerated the situation remarkably well and was in relatively good condition. Nevertheless, he was taken straight to the Resuscitaire by the waiting paediatricians and was brought back, pink, animated, and vigorously crying, to his relieved Mother within ten minutes of birth.

After a night of keeping Rose very busy breastfeeding, the baby was discharged home the next day in excellent health.

Debriefing and defusing fear: Catriona Cusick

The call buzzer went from the birthing room, I was being called as second midwife. On entering the room, I saw Ann in the pool in a semi-recumbent position with her baby's head delivered under the water, awaiting the next contraction. The lead midwife Sue told me the delivery of the head was two minutes ago and that restitution had not yet occurred (RCOG, 2012).

Sue informed me this was Ann's third baby and that although her two previous babies were large, she gave birth to them with no complication. Ann's contractions were frequent, hardly giving her a chance to catch her breath but she coped well, her husband Dan beside the pool supporting her.

Sue told me the basics that I needed to know about the labour so far during which the baby's head did not change position. Despite Ann's history of two normal births before, I felt slightly anxious. The absence of restitution was concerning me. I was anticipating the possibility of a shoulder dystocia.

Sue encouraged Ann to push with the next contraction and she did. I could see Ann was pushing with all her might. I slipped my hands into the water and gently felt to see if there was any movement of the baby's head, but there wasn't. I couldn't see any retraction of the baby's head (turtle-necking) (RCOG, 2012), and the baby's head didn't move. I looked at Sue hoping she would recognise the significance of this. We now needed to act quickly and skilfully without alarming Ann and her husband (RCOG, 2012).

In a split second, I asked Ann to stop pushing as it would only impact the shoulder further. I told her I was going to pull the emergency buzzer and that a few more people would arrive in the room. Looking into Ann 's eyes I spoke calmly to her, instructing her to get out of the pool straight away. As we carefully helped

Ann out of the pool, I guarded the baby's head with my hand. Another midwife, Helen, arrived, and I asked her to ring for the obstetric and neonatal teams to attend. Very shortly afterwards our maternity support worker Lou arrived, letting us know the Resuscitaire was ready. I was hoping that the manoeuvre of getting out of the pool would dislodge the baby's shoulders, allowing the baby to be born, but it had no effect.

I noticed Ann's husband looking extremely worried and scared. He removed himself to the corner of the room. Lou went over to him and I felt relieved to have her in the room helping. I gave him a reassuring nod and a smile. I wanted everyone to remain calm and although I could feel the adrenaline rushing through me, I knew that Sue and Helen would be feeling the same. Ann spontaneously went straight onto all fours and I started the internal manoeuvre of trying to deliver the posterior arm, but with no success. Sue and I looked at each other knowing that we had to move to the next manoeuvre immediately. We helped Ann to move onto her back and assisted her into the McRoberts' position (PROMPT, 2018). I could see slight movement of the baby's head and this gave me hope. I asked Sue to start suprapubic pressure, she located the baby's back and applied the appropriate pressure. Once again, I attempted to reach the posterior arm, but I was unsuccessful. Helen had come back into the room and helped Sue maintain Ann's legs in the McRoberts' position. She whispered in my ear that the obstetric teams were all in theatre but that the newborn team were on their way.

The adrenaline was coursing through my veins at this news, but I knew we needed to carry on with our manoeuvres and I also thought that Ann and Dan must extremely scared. I kept telling them what I was doing to keep them calm and to inform other midwives in the room helping me. I was the only one speaking though; there was stillness and a quietness that was unnerving.

I managed to reach the posterior arm and was able to deliver it. Relief flooded over me because I could feel the baby was coming. I had managed to dis-impact the shoulders and the baby was born, straightforwardly, after that. He was a big baby boy with very poor tone. It was exactly seven minutes from delivery of the baby's head to the birth of his body. He was not breathing and limp. Ann's husband cried, 'is he dead, what are you doing?!' Together with Helen, I started to resuscitate the baby, after giving an initial five inflation breaths, we saw good chest rise, so we were confident we had inflated the baby's lungs. The baby's heart rate was fast; his colour changed from blue to a reassuring pink and he tried to cry (Resuscitation Council (UK), 2015). I explained what was happening to Ann and Dan, trying my best to reassure them but Ann didn't say anything, she was lying there with her eyes closed and her husband was openly crying.

The newborn and obstetric teams arrived within seconds of each other and the noise levels increased dramatically. They were asking lots of necessary questions about the birth and subsequent events, but it changed the ambience in the room quite dramatically. However, once they could see the mother and baby were doing well, they soon left. I wanted to instil normality into what had been a shocking interlude in Ann and Dan's experience of birth, so I lifted the baby from the

Resuscitaire and took him over to Ann. She opened her arms and lovingly said, 'hello little man, so you're the one that's making all this trouble, are you?'

Ann looked at me and said 'I'm sorry, I just needed to close my eyes and listen to your instruction when all of that happened. I knew things were serious; I had to shut everything else out and just listen to your voice. I felt safe in your hands. I feel better now, I feel ok, thank you'.

I turned to see Ann's husband, who was now sitting with his head in his hands, adjusting to what had just happened. I went over to him and touched him on his shoulder, saying 'come on and meet your son'. We left the couple to enjoy their new arrival and to speak with each other privately for a few moments.

I immediately debriefed with the maternity staff involved, just to make sure everyone was okay. Sue told me that she had never seen a shoulder dystocia before. We discussed the importance of recognising the signs of a developing dystocia and of knowing the manoeuvres necessary to solve one. After our discussion, Sue told me that although it was frightening at the time, the experience had been invaluable as she had seen the manoeuvres performed in a real-life situation and that they had been successful.

I was also concerned about the couple. They had both been undoubtedly traumatised and I needed to address this in order to help them over their ordeal. I went back into the room and explained to Ann and Dan exactly what had happened, giving them the opportunity to tell me how they felt and to ask any questions they had. I made sure the room was decluttered of all the birth equipment, dirty linen, etc., found a comfortable place for Dan and me to sit next to Ann (and baby who was skin to skin and very happy) and got us all a cup of tea. Dan went through all his concerns and I listened to them intently. I answered all of Ann and Dan's questions calmly and logically in order to ensure that my explanations were clear and appropriate to aid their understanding. I also complimented my descriptions with a doll and pelvis in order to demonstrate the physiology of a shoulder dystocia. I showed them how the baby's shoulders become impacted and the significance of the manoeuvres that we performed in order to free them. I feel this debrief of events helped Ann and Dan enormously, as the next day they seemed much more light-hearted and relaxed. They were soon discharged home, mother and baby being fit and well. Sue and I received a thank you card from Ann a couple of weeks later, thanking us for everything we had done. It made me feel very happy that everything turned out well.

Shoulder dystocia: reading the signs right! Pat Hutson

Gemma, a mother of two girls, arrived on the unit, having thought her membranes had broken some three hours earlier. She hadn't yet started contracting and reported that the amniotic fluid had been clear and the baby had been moving well. On inspection of her pad, I confirmed that her membranes had indeed broken and gave her the information of what options were open to her (NICE, 2017b). She chose to wait 24 hours before any medical intervention. However, she was reluctant to go home as, not only did she live over 30 minutes' drive away, she had also organised childcare and didn't want to have to reorganise her plans. I suggested she went out for some breakfast as she hadn't eaten and to see what happened over the next couple of hours. If there had been no change during this time, my advice was to consider going home to rest. Gemma was happy with this plan, and I reassured her that if there were any concerns or changes, she could come back to the unit immediately.

Before leaving, I looked through her notes. It was documented that both of Gemma's previous deliveries had been vaginal, with the first one being a ventouse-assisted birth. Baby number one had weighed 4390 g and baby two had weighed 4615 g. This pregnancy, her fundus measured 43 cm and the 34/40 ultrasound scan (USS) had put both the abdominal circumference and the biparietal circumference above the 95th centile. She went to see her consultant for the individual planning of her third labour and delivery, and to discuss mode and place of birth in view of her babies' weights (NICE, 2017a). After discussion, Gemma chose to be in our unit, as she wanted to use the pool (OUH, 2016)

Gemma was off the ward for a couple of hours when her partner rang in to say that the contractions had started, and Gemma felt she wanted my support as she had now begun to labour. Ten minutes later, when Gemma arrived on the unit for the second time, she appeared completely different from when I first met her. She was contracting regularly and having to concentrate to breathe through them. They were lasting around 45 secs and moderate on palpation. Her partner, Mark, commented that they had been at this level for over 30 minutes. As Gemma wanted to use the pool, I took her into a delivery room and began running the water whilst I carried out the usual observations (NICE, 2018a). During the 20 or so minutes this took, it was obvious that Gemma was in established labour and so I began normal first stage intrapartum care (NICE, 2018a).

As a rule, when a woman wants to use the pool, I explain that during the actual birth, it is important that the baby remains under the water until the whole of its body is born and that if she is asked to vacate the pool, it is paramount that she does so immediately. Gemma agreed and once the pool was ready, I invited Gemma to get in which she readily did.

Gemma was breathing through the contractions and then joining in the conversations with Mark and myself between them, but after being in the pool for some 40 minutes Gemma's behaviour changed. She became very quiet and ceased joining in the conversations. It was obvious she was having to concentrate to cope with the now strong contractions and occasionally she sounded expulsive. She requested Entonox which I provided, explaining how to use it to the best effect (NICE, 2018c).

As Gemma was now using the Entonox, the expulsive sound ceased, and Gemma reported she felt back in control of the situation and her body. A further 25 minutes passed, when suddenly Gemma pushed hard during a contraction and, on inspection of the pool water, I could see she had opened her bowels during this mighty contraction. This happened during the next three contractions and I could see external signs that delivery was now imminent. Over the next five minutes, the perineum flattened and the vertex became visible. However, the vertex advanced very slowly. I was somehow feeling uneasy with the slow descent of the head. Gradually, the baby's head began to crown. As this happened very slowly, I had alarm bells in my head, 'this was not what I would expect for a woman who had two vaginal births before!' However, in the back of my mind were the previous babies' weights and the ultrasound results. After a further three contractions, the head went from crowning to being born. At this point, I buzzed for a colleague to come into the room. I was strongly suspecting a shoulder dystocia was about to occur (RCOG, 2012).

With the next contraction, the head 'turtle-necked' and my suspicions grew even stronger! Calmly, I asked Gemma to leave the pool and get on the bed, explaining that I was concerned about the birth of the shoulders. Gemma, as asked, got straight out of the pool. I was mindful that standing and lifting one leg over the edge of the pool is often enough to free the shoulders, so I made sure that my hands were poised in case the baby delivered before we got to the bed. Unfortunately, this time, this did not happen, and Gemma got onto the bed into an all fours position. Whilst all this was happening, I asked my colleague to pull the emergency buzzer to ensure more people arrived to help. As it had now been two and a half minutes since the head had been delivered, an emergency call for the obstetric and paediatric team to attend was also put out. Gemma pushed once more, and the head did not move or rotate.

Once on the bed, the shoulder dystocia protocol was started. I asked Gemma not to push and try to breathe through the next contraction whilst we helped her to move onto her back. Gemma's legs were put into the McRoberts' position (RCOG, 2012), hoping that this manoeuvre would facilitate the birth of the baby's shoulders, but this was to no avail. A quick abdominal palpation told us that the foetal back was on maternal left and one of my colleagues began suprapubic pressure (RCOG, 2012). This didn't work either. Therefore, I began internal manoeuvres (RCOG, 2012). Worryingly, I was unable to feel the posterior arm. 'Okay, I have to go further', I told myself. And I did. I located the arm pit and by tracing my way down to the elbow, I managed to grab the wrist and bring the hand over the baby's face, thus releasing the shoulder. This had all taken a further two and a half minutes, during which time both emergency teams had arrived. Once the shoulder had been released, delivery of the rest of the body followed easily. It had taken almost six minutes between the birth of the head and body. The big baby boy was white and floppy after the birth and after tactile stimulation (Resuscitation Council (UK), 2016) remained limp and pale. With the help of my colleague, we quickly dried the baby, put a hat on, and changed the towel for a dry one to keep him warm. I requested the bag and mask and proceeded to do five inflation breaths (Resuscitation Council (UK), 2016). On the third inflation breath, the lungs were seen to be inflated and at 30 seconds when reassessing (Resuscitation Council (UK), 2016) the heart rate, which had been under 100 beats per minute (bpm), now rose to over 120 bpm. After a further round of ventilation breaths, the baby began to gasp under the mask, and then let out a hearty cry. I think I am not wrong by saying that, at that point, everybody in the room breathed again with utter relief. The baby was put skin to skin with mum and I continued to manage the third stage of labour. A full debriefing was carried out later that day with the couple and all their questions on what had happened answered. The baby weighed an impressive 5010 g!

Shoulder dystocia and a language barrier, a midwife's frightening journey: Maria Paz Miranda

It was handover time at the end of my day shift. It was summer and we were commenting about the need of getting an ice machine to provide our women with cold water for the summer ahead. Lucy, one of the women in labour that night, was in the pool and approaching the second stage of labour of her second child. At handover, my colleague verbalised her concerns about the little English spoken by her and the family. She advised the night staff to call an interpreter to make sure that Lucy was able to understand and consent to the procedures (NICE, 2010). A third-year student was with Lucy during handover, with the expressed instructions to call us straight away in case of any worries or concerns.

The handover happened smoothly and without any incidents to report.

I entered the changing room feeling relaxed and already disconnected from what was happening in the labour ward. I made a few phone calls and changed my blue scrubs for my favourite jeans. It was 19:50 on a lovely warm evening. I was leaving the unit, at the door, when I heard the emergency buzzer. That noise, too well known, put me instantly on guard. Looking at the illuminated board in the middle of the corridor, identifying the room, and running towards it only took me a few seconds.

As I entered the room, I saw Lucy in the pool, on her back, floating. She was conscious and alert, looking petite in the middle of the big pool. My mind was racing: the water was clear, so it was not a postpartum haemorrhage or an antepartum haemorrhage. There was not significant meconium either. Then, I saw my colleague with her arms in the water; however, I did not see the baby. Just the head had been born. A second midwife was standing by the pool, urging Lucy to abandon the pool quickly. The student was standing in a corner and our night maternity support worker was by the desk, documenting the events in the maternity notes. The family was in the other corner of the room, looking frightened. The atmosphere in the room had that feeling of coldness and quietness.

Both midwives shouted at the same time: shoulder dystocia! (RCOG, 2012).

I felt the clock ticking in my head. How many minutes since the birth of the head? I asked in the calmest voice I could find. 'Three minutes' they answered. They had documented the time. What's next? I asked myself, trying to put my thoughts in order. I asked again, about how many pushes since the delivery of the head. My colleague told me that Lucy had pushed once since the delivery of the head.

Our next task was to persuade Lucy, in the strongest possible terms, to evacuate the pool. But she did not respond to our request. Was she understanding our instructions? Could she move? Was something else impeding her movement? Did she want to move? After a few seconds, a third midwife arrived to help.

We decided to intervene in a more active way. Two midwives supported Lucy by her armpits; our aim was to guide her, physically, to abandon the pool. Believe me, it is a very difficult task to achieve. Lucy was not cooperating, and her dead weight was too much for the two midwives bending over the edges of the pool when they tried to help her stand up.

Then she had another contraction. My colleagues helped her to stand, adopting a leaning forwards position in the pool this time. She pushed. Her baby's head did not show any signs of the reassuring external rotation or restitution of the head, hoped and expected (RCOG, 2012). We were in serious trouble. We needed extra help. I asked our maternity support worker, Sophie, to put an emergency call for the obstetric and neonatal team to attend and help us with the shoulder dystocia in development. One of the midwives took the role of scriber as the situation become more complex. Sophie was asked by my colleague to take care of the family.

I inquired how many minutes again since the birth of the head. Our efforts were against the clock. Five minutes now since the delivery of the head. Somehow, we managed to get Lucy to stay up, walk towards the end of the pool, and after a great effort, evacuate it.

In the middle of the room she had another contraction and an unbearable urge to push. We could not stop her from pushing, it was hard for her to listen to our instructions. The language barrier was taking its toll. We guided her towards the floor, in an 'all fours' position (RCOG, 2012; Shiers, 1999). As she pushed, I was kneeling by her side, but no changes were seen. the baby's head did not rotate. We did not touch or apply any traction. It was futile. We knew that those shoulders had not rotated internally. Gently but firmly, we helped her to walk towards the bed and to assume an all fours position, this time on the bed. Our plan was to try an all fours position for the second time and then ask her to move onto her back to perform the McRoberts' manoeuvre (RCOG, 2012; Shiers, 1999; Coates, 1995). Why all fours first? Because I was sure that if we tried McRoberts first, Lucy wouldn't move to try 'all fours' after being on her back.

As soon as she adopted the all fours position on the bed, I saw the head slowly rotating towards the right. When I saw the head rotating, I felt incredibly relieved. I knew that the shoulders had been rotating internally and possibly disengaged themselves from the position assumed before. The short walk towards the bed did the trick! With the next push, I applied light, axial, routine traction (RCOG, 2012), following the curve of the pelvis (remember the posterior part of the pelvis is now is facing me). I felt the shoulders being delivered. I saw the posterior shoulder slowly appearing under the perineum with my own eyes. An incredible sensation of relief invaded me. As I was delivering the baby, the obstetric and neonatal emergency team arrived.

The baby was born without tone and almost white eight minutes after the delivery of the head.

With the paediatric doctor by my side, following her advice, and as the baby's heart rate was over 100 bpm, we decided to wait to allow the baby to take advantage from the uncut cord, benefiting from the blood still being pumped to the baby (Wyllie et al., 2015). At 30 seconds, the baby's heart rate was increasing, very reassuring. At the same time, Syntometrine intramuscular was given to Lucy, to prevent a postpartum haemorrhage associated with this emergency (RCOG, 2012). Around 50 seconds after delivery of the body, the baby was getting some colour back in her body, she was attempting to move her limbs but was unable to breathe regularly. The heartbeat was above 100 bpm when the neonatal doctor auscultated it. The cord was clamped and cut at 1 minute of life, and the baby girl was passed to the paediatric doctor and one of my colleagues. They initiated resuscitation manoeuvres without any delay. Lucy was crying. My colleague was holding Lucy's hand with a tender look in her eyes, a gesture that means more than a thousand spoken words. During the whole emergency, she had been speaking with Lucy, explaining what was happening, reassuring her, gently touching her, caressing her, letting her know about the next move. It was hard for her as Lucy spoke little English. It took us a few moments to compose ourselves. Within a couple of minutes, everybody had a role to play.

The placenta was delivered without any incident and normal blood loss occurred. Lucy had sustained a perineal trauma that was promptly sutured. The neonatal doctor was the busiest one in the team. The baby was struggling to maintain her airways open and needed assisted ventilation. However, after a few ventilation breaths, the baby could breathe on her own and started to grunt. She was transferred to the neonatal unit for observation and potential further treatment. Before the transfer, the baby was weighed, two labels identifying the baby were placed on her ankles, and vitamin K intramuscular was discussed with the parents. They accepted and consented to it (Knight, 2014). We encouraged the father to accompany the baby to the intensive care unit, but he declined; he wanted to stay with his wife.

I washed my shaking hands and headed off to the office to complete the Shoulder Dystocia Form. My colleague had taken very good and contemporaneous records of the events, with the times of every manoeuvre and the staff involved in them; therefore, completing the form was easy. My next task was to recall the traumatic events with Lucy and her husband, allowing enough time to ask questions and help them to understand the nature of the emergency just experienced by the whole family. I started the conversation by offering an interpreter. However, they told me that if we spoke slowly, they could understand and felt confident that they could ask every question that they considered pertinent.

Before I left the unit, Sophie prepared the loveliest cup of tea imaginable for me! I drank it, called my husband, apologising as he had been waiting for me downstairs, in our car since 20:00 hours.

Learning points

Shoulder dystocia, and whether it is a preventable event, is a matter for heated discussion. We invite you to join in the discussion by sharing with you our reflections derived from our experiences of shoulder dystocia in the pool. We have separated them into the following categories.

Before the emergency

- Familiarise yourself with the mechanics of birth. It will allow you to diagnose any abnormality.
- Regular skills and drills sessions are an ongoing and essential part of learning and development for all of us.
- Know your manoeuvres well, you have time to perform them. Even the most experienced midwives find this emergency very stressful, it not just you.
- Be aware of the risk factors. For example: ⇧ BMI, previous large baby, slow progress in first and/or second stage of labour, high head in the intrapartum period, instrumental delivery.
- Always be prepared for a speedy exit from the pool, discuss it with the woman in advance.

During the emergency

- Call for help immediately. Summon the obstetric team and the newborn team.
- State the emergency with clarity and without hesitation: I think this is a shoulder dystocia.
- Stay calm. It will allow you to think about the best course of action.
- Assign a scriber. Precise and timely documentation is vital.
- Assign someone to reassure the family, keep them informed all the time.
- Speak clearly, state manoeuvre and time.
- Advise the woman not to push whilst you are performing manoeuvres.
- Do not apply traction until you are sure that the shoulders have rotated internally.

After the emergency

- Complete shoulder dystocia proforma as part of an audit process that will enable future improvements in practice.
- Have a structured debriefing with the woman, birth companion, and all staff involved in the emergency. Reflect on the events. Write up your own personal reflection to consolidate your learning.

References

Coates, T., 1995. Shoulder dystocia. In: J. Alexander, V. Levy & S. Roch, eds. *Aspects of Midwifery Practice: A Research-Based Approach*, 1st edition. London: Macmillan, p. 80.

Coates, T., 1997. Shoulder dystocia. In: B. Sweet & D. Tiran, eds. *Mayes' Midwifery: A Textbook for Midwives*, 12th edition. Edinburgh: Bailliere Tindall, pp. 661–668.

Knight, L., 2014. Oxford University Hospitals Trust. [Online] Available at: www.ouh. nhs.uk/patient-guide/leaflets/files/10711Pvitamink.pdf [Accessed 15 November 2017].

Morrin, N. A., 1997. Midwifery care in the second stage of labour. In: B. Sweet & D. Tiran, eds. *Mayes' Midwifery: A Textbook for Midwives*, 12th edition. Edinburgh: Bailliere Tindall, p. 398.

NICE, 2010. Enhance care delivery for pregnant women, with complex social factors, help women who have difficulty reading or speaking English to communicate. Information and support. NICE guideline CG110. [Online] Available at: https://pathways.nice.org.uk/pathways/pregnancy-and-complex-social-factors-service-provision#path=view%3A/pathways/pregnancy-and-complex-social-factors-service-provision/pregnant-women-who-are-recent-migrants-asylum-seekers-or-refugees-or-have-difficulty [Accessed 1 September 2017].

NICE, 2017a. Intrapartum care for healthy women and babies. NICE Guidelines [CG190]. Place of birth. [Online] Available at: www.nice.org.uk/guidance/cg190/chapter/Recommendations#place-of-birth [Accessed 17 July 2018].

NICE, 2017b. Intrapartum care for healthy women and babies. NICE Guidelines [CG190]. Prelabour rupture of membranes at term. [Online] Available at: www.nice.org.uk/guidance/cg190/chapter/Recommendations#prelabour-rupture-of-membranes-at-term [Accessed 6 August 2018].

NICE, 2018a. Care in established first stage of labour. [Online] Available at: https://pathways.nice.org.uk/pathways/intrapartum-care#path=view%3A/pathways/intrapartum-care/care-in-established-first-stage-of-labour.xml&content=view-index [Accessed 3 March 2018].

NICE, 2018b. Care in second stage of labour. [Online] Available at: https://pathways.nice.org.uk/pathways/intrapartum-care#path=view%3A/pathways/intrapartum-care/care-in-second-stage-of-labour.xml&content=view-index [Accessed 3 March 2018].

NICE, 2018c. Pain relief in labour. [Online] Available at: https://pathways.nice.org.uk/pathways/intrapartum-care/pain-relief-in-labour#content=view-node%3Anodes-non-pharmacological-and-inhalational-analgesia [Accessed 29 January 2018].

OUH, 2016. Birth choices in Oxfordshire. [Online] Available at: www.ouh.nhs.uk/patient-guide/leaflets/files/13511Pbirth.pdf [Accessed 7 July 2018].

PROMPT, 2018. Shoulder dystocia training. [Online] Available at: www.youtube.com/channel/UCh8PZGugxqDKBUcpTrulAfw [Accessed 29 January 2018].

RCOG, 2012. Royal College of Obstetricians and Gynaecologists. *Shoulder Dystocia. Green – Top Guideline No. 42*, 2nd edition. [Online] Available at: www.rcog.org.uk/globalassets/documents/guidelines/gtg_42.pdf [Accessed 21 November 2017].

Resuscitation Council (UK), 2015. The guideline process. [Online] Available at: www.resus.org.uk/resuscitation-guidelines/resuscitation-and-support-of-transition-of-babies-at-birth/#process [Accessed 18 April 2018].

Resuscitation Council (UK), 2016. *New Born Life Support*, 4th edition. London: Resuscitation Council (UK).

Shiers, C. V., 1999. Midwifery and obstetric emergencies. Shoulder dystocia. In: R. Bennet & L. Brown, eds. *Myles' Midwifery: A Text for Midwives*, 13th edition. Edinburgh: Churchill Livingstone, p. 569.

Stables, D., 1999. Cephalopelvic disproportion, obstructed labour and other obstetric emergencies. In: D. Stables, ed. *Physiology in Childbearing with Anatomy and Related Biosciences*. Edinburgh: Harcourt Publishers Ltd, pp. 529–530.

Wyllie, J., Ainsworth, S., & Tinnion, R., 2015. Important guideline changes. In: J. Wyllie, S. Ainsworth & R. Tinnion, eds. *Resuscitation and support of transition of babies at birth*. London: Resuscitation Council (UK). [Online] Available at: www.resus.org.uk/resuscitation-guidelines/resuscitation-and-support-of-transition-of-babies-at-birth/#changes [Accessed 14 December 2017].

Chapter 6

Unexpected events in the water

Maria Paz Miranda, Sian Marie Barnard, Catriona Cusick, and Pat Hutson

Introduction

Women labouring and birthing in a midwifery-led unit expect their labour will progress without any serious incidents or complications. Consequently, any disruption of those expectations is not good news at all. We work very hard to keep a labouring woman within normal parameters: we are attentive to factors such as mobilisation, bladder care, drinking and eating sensibly, and we are vigilant to maternal and foetal wellbeing. To achieve this, we use our theoretical and practical knowledge accumulated during the years of experience working in a low-risk setting, with clear boundaries and guidelines. However, unexpected events will continue to happen. We endeavour to find a fine balance between safety and respecting the woman's birthing choices within a low-risk environment. This is central to our philosophy – what we do and how do we do it will surely impact on the overall perception of the birthing experience (RCM, 2012c).

These stories are based on real-life experiences. The confidentiality of the women has been protected, however, these accounts describe the actual management of unexpected clinical situations that have challenged our practice in the pool, in real time, as experienced by us. Our intention is to show how we dealt with these unexpected events, trying to keep the disruption of the normal process of labour and birth to a minimum whilst at the same time providing care that is evidence based, safe, and in accordance with our local hospital and NICE guidelines.

We hope that the reader finds these narratives interesting and useful in their own clinical practice. To make it more relevant, we have included our personal reflections at the end of the chapter, which, we hope, will encourage further discussion.

Maternal sepsis: Sian Marie Barnard

Katie was so happy to have arrived on the unit, in established labour, to find the delivery room of her choice was available. Ever since she had attended the 36-week tour of the unit, she had her heart fixed on the light sensory suite. She had instantly felt the room had a feeling of warmth, tranquillity, and cosiness.

In addition to this, and most important of all, was the inclusion of a pool! This was Katie's third pregnancy and she so hoped to have a waterbirth. Her other two children were born in mainland Europe, where the use of water in labour had not been available to her. Her husband's work had brought her and her family to the UK during this pregnancy and Katie had researched the possibility of using water for her labour. During the tour, she was overjoyed to discover the pool would be an available option for her to use this time.

Katie's labour was progressing well. On assessment, all maternal and foetal observations were normal (NICE, 2017f) and I found her cervix to be 4 cm dilated and fully effaced. I had begun to run the pool after her initial phone call, so it was nearly full and ready for use by the time I had performed the assessment. Katie's contractions were regular and strong (NICE, 2017f), but she was coping beautifully with them. Her breathing technique was slow and controlled; she seemed focused and practical. Katie's husband and I gathered up all their bags and paraphernalia and the three of us made our way down the corridor heading towards the much-anticipated light sensory pool room. Only a gentle light illuminated the corner of the room and the tranquil lilac, turquoise, and soft pink lights bathed the rest of the space. As she walked in, Katie commented on the warm, soothing ambience and enthused about how happy she was to be in the room that she had fixated on four weeks previously.

The pool looked so inviting; it took on the lovely soothing hues of the unicorn-coloured sensory lighting. Katie changed into her specially chosen 'labour' bikini and got in. Her husband smiled with satisfaction because Katie had realised her goal of labouring in water. The contractions continued with unceasing rhythm and strength. They continued to gain momentum in the following few hours, but Katie rose to the challenge as she moved from kneeling and leaning forwards to resting and leaning back against the side of the pool, submerging her abdomen under the water, maximising its supportive, weight-relieving qualities (Garland, 2011a). I kept the pool temperature constant at 37°C (NICE, 2014), as Katie found most comfort in the water being as warm as it could safely be. Over the next few hours, Katie's labour progressed smoothly, her baby girl was active in utero. Katie could feel her baby's head 'moving down' when the contractions were at their height. The foetal heart rate was reassuring (NICE, 2017), and the atmosphere in the room was tranquil as Katie moved around freely in the water, spontaneously adopting the kind of positions that are conducive to a normal birth with ease (Garland, 2011a; Burns, 2004). Katie seemed to be in tune with her body; it was as if being immersed in the deep, temperate water within the privacy of the cosy, quiet room was exactly the kind of primordial environment she craved.

By the time of the next vaginal examination four hours later, Katie's cervix was 8 cm dilated; normal progress had been made. The baby's head was in an optimal occipital anterior position and at −1 to the ischial spines (Sweet, 1997a). Maternal observations were normal (NICE, 2017); the clinical picture looked good. Katie was pleased with these findings and keen to get straight back in the pool. The solace Katie found when in the warm, incandescent water was tangible.

About half an hour later, Katie started to feel nauseous. She then suddenly vomited up all the fluid she had been drinking over the last couple of hours. This is not an uncommon reaction when contractions are strong and powerful, but given Katie's previous calmness and honed breathing technique, I was a little surprised this happened. After she had caught her breath and recovered, she told me she felt very tired.

An abrupt and very noticeable change in Katie's demeanour then followed. Her previous convivial attitude had changed; she rapidly became much more withdrawn, almost distant, and her contractions also began to space and out and diminish. I considered that this might be due to the transition of labour (Kitzinger, 2000), so I just continued to observe, monitor, and reassure, but looking back, I felt a sense of slight apprehension and uncertainty about the dramatic 'shift' in Katie's behaviour.

Within a short while, Katie then told me she felt cold. This concerned me. I was not expecting her to feel cold given the pool temperature was 36.9°C, the room was warm, humid in fact, and draught free. She was tired yes, but only 40 minutes or so before this, her contractions had been regular and strong, causing her to flush and perspire. Now Katie was pale and listless, and her labour had not just abated, but ebbed away. My suspicions were raised, this was not normal. I proceeded to check Katie's temperature with a tympanic thermometer; it read 38.1°C. I felt Katie's forehead, she felt warm, but not feverish. Her pulse was 64 bpm and her blood pressure was 116/62, her respiratory rate was also within the normal range (NICE, 2017).

Really ... a temperature of 38.1°C, I thought? This pyrexia seemed to have sprung up from nowhere. There were no risk factors for sepsis, yet this appeared to be what we were faced with. I checked her temperature again ... still 38.1°C, then again with the oral thermometer, it recorded 38.2°C. I also checked my own temperature with the same thermometer, just to be sure ... it read 36.9°C. There was no doubt, Katie had developed sepsis and I needed to act swiftly.

I knew that this meant Katie's labour care would now deviate away from using the pool that was working so well for her. Unfortunately, the ambience would now need to be disturbed and Katie's labour journey would take another direction, leading her away from the waterbirth she had wanted. I was crushed for her, but I could not delay the necessary actions that needed to follow in order to manage the sepsis effectively. Time was now of the essence, so despite the undoubted anxiety and disappointment leaving the water would bring, this was what I needed to advise Katie to do.

I explained the significance of the pyrexia to Katie and that we would need to transfer to the consultant-led unit (CLU) immediately for activation of the sepsis protocol (RCOG, 2017).

Katie stood up to get out of the pool without delay, but as she did so, the emotional and physical wrench of having to leave the water was so overwhelming for her that she began to cry. She understood and accepted the need for transfer but was also hugely frustrated and upset that her own body had denied her the waterbirth she had so longed for; her disappointment was palpable.

Although the situation was serious, and Katie needed immediate treatment, it was important for me to try to maintain a positive atmosphere and remain composed. I wanted Katie to feel as untroubled as possible by the impending introduction of monitors, drips, and blood tests that would ensue following our transfer. I reassured Katie that despite the necessary interventions and procedures involved in the sepsis protocol (RCOG, 2017), she still needed to focus on the joy of meeting her beautiful new baby. I assured her that once on the CLU, we would commence telemetry in order that she would still be able to freely move unhindered by cardiotocography machine leads, and that we could have a diffuser in the room with harmonising chamomile and lavender essential oils to enhance relaxation. I also explained that once all necessary procedures to manage the sepsis had been actioned, we could lower the lighting in order to promote a calming atmosphere and subsequent oxytocin release (Kitzinger, 2000).

Just as we were preparing to leave, my colleague informed me that we were unable to transfer immediately as the next available room on the CLU was still being cleaned. So, whilst we waited, I used the extra few minutes to site a cannula in Katie's left forearm and obtained the bloods required for the sepsis protocol (RCOG, 2017) in order that they could be sent urgently in advance. I also asked my colleague to request that the necessary antibiotics be prescribed and drawn up in preparation for our arrival. I checked Katie's observations again and documented them accordingly onto the observations chart. Katie was now developing a tachycardia; her resting heart rate was 104 bpm, her blood pressure had fallen to 90/48 mmHg, and her respiratory rate had risen to 21 pm. These were all symptoms of a systemic inflammatory response syndrome (SIRS); in view of this, I commenced intravenous fluids immediately to help counteract the hypotension (RCOG, 2017).

Within one hour of the diagnosis, Katie was on the CLU, sepsis protocol actioned; broad spectrum intravenous antibiotics had been administered (RCOG, 2017) and a cardiotocograph (with telemetry) was in progress and looking reassuring. Katie responded well to the treatment and her contractions later re-established. Although there was no evidence of foetal distress, I ensured a paediatrician was present for the birth in case of the need for neonatal resuscitation – I anticipated that the sepsis may have caused a biochemical disturbance in the baby that would interfere with the normal physiology of transition at birth (Wylie et al., 2016a). I was also aware that in the event of a potential low haemoglobin level (caused by the sepsis), the risk of a postpartum haemorrhage increases; therefore, I equipped my delivery trolley accordingly and I gained consent from Katie for Syntometrine to be administered with the birth of the baby's anterior shoulder in order to actively manage the third stage of labour (NICE, 2017g). I also made sure a second midwife was present for the birth and that I had immediate access to an obstetrician should it become necessary. Thankfully, Katie gave birth to her baby daughter without complication and the newborn observations were completely normal (NICE, 2012). Katie went home the next day on a course of oral antibiotics and both she and her baby were in good health; testament to the early diagnosis and prompt treatment of maternal sepsis.

Waiting for the reassuring cry! Sian Marie Barnard

I had only just been recently reflecting on how babies often seem more relaxed following a pool birth and how those babies born in the water often don't cry immediately (Walsh, 2012b). In relation to this, a matter of interest to me has always been how to know when the absence of a cry is normal and when it is not. What evidence do we have for this? There a fine line between a newly born baby not crying because it's in a relaxed, non-stressed state and a baby that is not crying because it is compromised in some way.

To hear a cry immediately after birth is often a very reassuring sign of wellbeing for parents. So how do we differentiate between the need for passive observation and the need to intervene? How do we gain the confidence to wait and reassure the parents that everything is okay?

It is well known that the important physiological processes necessary for adaptation to extrauterine respiration occur in the neonate during those first precious minutes following birth (Coad & Dunstall, 2001). This period of 'transition' is also a time when optimal hormonal conditions exist for bonding a mother and her baby (Walsh, 2012a). Therefore, the importance of leaving mother and baby undisturbed during this time is obvious and is a philosophy to which waterbirth naturally inclines. However, this story demonstrates that if a baby is unable to cry, he is at the mercy of those caring for him to recognise that he is compromised and needs attention.

I was introduced to Chloe whilst she was in the pool in the second stage of labour birthing her first baby. She had made excellent progress from the diagnosis of established labour only six hours previously. Chloe was calm and composed and was able to engage with me warmly despite being in strong labour. Her partner Steve was also pleasant and relaxed. Handover was swift and succinct. Chloe had experienced a straightforward pregnancy and it appeared she was heading nicely towards a normal physiological birth.

Chloe's waters had broken an hour previously and were reported as clear. Indeed, when I looked down into the pool, I could see flecks of white vernix on the surface of the water and some bloody mucousy show on the bottom of the pool. I could see that the liquor seeping occasionally from the introitus was clear. The foetal heart rate baseline was reported to have been 140 bpm to this point – accelerations had been heard and no decelerations were reported (NICE, 2017). Chloe was kneeling and leaning forwards in the water, and there were obvious external signs that indicated the vertex was soon likely to be visible (Morrin, 1997a). Chloe seemed completely unphased by the apparent immanency of the birth; with the next contraction she just 'breathed through' with a naturalness and intuitiveness that was lovely to see. I lowered my angled mirror down into the water to enable me to visualise the perineum and yes, I could see vertex, just visible. What an amazing woman; this was such good progress.

As Chloe's second stage of labour advanced, the foetal heart rate remained reassuring, she began to respond to the surges of pressure with a subtle bearing down and within 20 minutes of this behaviour, the vertex was approaching crowning.

Although Chloe was doing remarkably well, it was important for me to provide guidance during the birth of the baby's head. Just by offering gentle verbal support, I encouraged her to follow her body's natural urges and to try to breathe through the crowning phase to allow the perineal tissue to stretch gradually (Morrin, 1997a). Only now did Chloe feel overwhelmed by the intense stretching and burning sensation she was feeling; I encouraged her to just 'breathe' through it if she could. Chloe rose to the challenge, and she mustered her resolve and managed to focus beautifully. The baby's head was born with natural momentum and restitution occurred a few moments afterwards (Morrin, 1997a; Hillan, 1999). The next contraction followed just two minutes later; as it was building, I could see the nape of the baby's neck advancing forwards, then with the next surge, a steady push from Chloe resulted in a serene waterbirth. I circled my hands around the baby's body and moved him upwards in a gentle emergence to the surface of the water.

The cord was long enough to allow Chloe to have her baby cuddled up against her chest without undue cord tension preventing any potential of snapping (Garland, 2011b). The baby was pink, with normal tone and his heart rate was above 100 bpm. He began to open his eyes and he was breathing normally (Wylie et al., 2016). I was happy to leave the cord pulsating to allow its perfusion to naturally oxygenate him. I had in mind that the transitional physiology of the waterbirth baby can be different to that of a baby born on dry land (Garland, 2011b) and therefore I needed to allow a true minute for an honest and accurate Apgar reading.

At one minute of age, I gave the baby an Apgar score of 8 (NICE, 2017a). He hadn't cried, but his colour was pink, his heart rate was above 120 bpm, his body had tone but he was not moving, and I could see he was breathing regularly; he appeared to be 'transitioning' normally (Wylie et al., 2016). I continued to watch him carefully though, waiting for the reassuring cry that would assure me all was well with him. Chloe was cradling the baby so that his body was totally submerged under the water this was keeping him nice and warm.

By two minutes of age his cry still hadn't come, but I didn't want to unnecessarily disturb the ambience just yet (NICE, 2017a). This baby's calm disposition meant that I wasn't overly surprised he hadn't cried immediately. All the other signs of wellbeing were present (Wylie et al., 2016), so I was happy to wait a little longer. Another minute passed, and I was still watching and waiting for a cry. The baby's eyes were open and all the other observations of him were normal, but I was just becoming a little concerned that he wasn't progressing into more reassuring, active behaviour as I would have expected by this point. Chloe and Steve were stroking his arms and talking to him, and though on the face of it things 'looked' normal, I couldn't help but feel uneasy. My holistic assessment of the baby was telling me that I needed to persist in waiting for the cry.

I decided to try and initiate this by just lifting him up out of the water with the cord still attached. Most babies don't like this, and they'll show their annoyance by giving you a yell! Although I didn't want to disturb Chloe's special bonding time, I did want to hear a cry from this baby. I felt by intervening in this minor way, I could illicit a response that would reassure me he was okay.

As I held him, suspended just above the surface of the water, he grimaced and drew his arms and legs inwards and started to cry … 'that's what I was waiting for' I said and placed him back into Chloe's arms; still watching and waiting for a full-blown holler!

But it didn't come; instead, over the next few moments the baby's colour faded from pink to a pale greyish hue and his previous normal tone changed to limp and floppy. His eyes were still open, but they were just staring into space, vacant and dark. He literally just 'went off' in front of my eyes. I quickly explained to Chloe that I needed to clamp and cut the cord straight away and take the baby over to the bed in order that I would have a dry flat surface to assess him properly. I asked the maternity support worker already in the room to summon the second midwife immediately, then to emergency call the neonatal team, switch on the Resuscitaire, and report back to me once all this was done. I proceeded to wipe the baby vigorously with a dry towel, put a clean, dry hat on him, and wrap him with more towels leaving only his chest uncovered. This enabled me to properly assess his colour, tone breathing, and heart rate (Wylie et al., 2016).

The baby was now breathing irregularly and showing signs of respiratory distress (Wylie et al., 2016). I could see chest recession and nasal flaring; he was struggling. His heart rate was 160 bpm. This baby needed help.

The second midwife arrived and retrieved the bag and mask. I positioned the baby ready to administer ventilation breaths (Wylie et al., 2016). With the first and second inflations, I couldn't see any chest rise. It is so important to stay calm and logical if the first attempt at administering inflation or ventilation breaths doesn't work, and this is exactly what I told myself. I repositioned the baby's head, and then repositioned the face mask, and we tried again. This time, I saw a clear 'rise 'in the baby's chest and from the next ventilation breath, he 'pinked up' nicely. This was a good response and reassurance that we were achieving our aim of oxygenating the baby (Wylie et al., 2016). At five minutes of age, I gave the baby an Apgar score of 6 (NICE, 2017a); he was pink, but limp, breathing irregularly and still only grimacing. Just at this moment, the door opened, and the newborn team arrived. I gave them a succinct handover of events and they proceeded to take over and manage the care of the baby from this point. He was immediately taken to the Resuscitaire for continued ventilation breaths and a comprehensive clinical assessment of his condition (NICE, 2017a).

Chloe and Steve were obviously shocked and extremely anxious. I tried to soothe them by explaining that the baby's condition was stable and that he was in expert hands; however, I also had to be honest in letting her know the situation was serious (NMC, 2015). I informed Chloe that her baby would need continued clinical investigation to isolate the cause of his compromise and the appropriate treatment to help resolve it (Simpson, 1997). I ensured the information I gave her was objective and that I avoided prejudging the care the neonatal team would need to give (Wylie et al., 2016). The maternity support worker kindly offered to accompany Chloe's partner to see and be with the baby whilst the paediatricians were caring for him. This would hopefully help him to feel more connected and involved. He could also then report back to Chloe, keeping her updated on their baby's condition until she was able to join them. I later learnt that the baby had a septic screen and went home after having a course of intravenous antibiotics. His cultures showed group B streptococcus was present (RCOG, 2017).

I am so glad that I was alert to this baby's compromise that day and that my colleagues and I took the necessary steps to manage his deteriorating condition promptly and effectively. It was the absence of 'the reassuring cry' that led me to recognise that something wasn't quite right.

The fourth-degree tear: Catriona Cusick

I first met Annie and Mick when I was relieving the community midwife for her lunch break. The couple were having their first baby. Annie was in the first stage of labour and she had not long got into the pool. Annie seemed to be finding the pool beneficial. The community midwife went on to describe how Annie was finding that the water was easing her backache and generally helping her to cope with the intensity of her contractions. I could see the buoyancy of the water gave her the freedom to mobilise without restraint (Cluett & Burns, 2009). Mick was also in the pool I could see that he was fully engaged and wanting to be close with Annie every step of the way. Annie and I fell into easy conversation and found that we shared a love of ballroom dancing and my time with them both passed very quickly!

I left the room on the community midwife's return, secretly hoping to be called as second midwife in order to be able to witness Annie's lovely waterbirth.

A little later I was called back to the room, Annie was now in active second stage. Everything appeared fine. Then, I glanced down towards Annie's perineum; I could see the baby's head advancing, but something didn't look quite right. It took me several seconds to comprehend what I was visualising. The perineum was bulging, and I could see vertex was visible at the introitus, but also, I could see vertex through the dilated anal opening.

My brain was stalling, I was thinking what? … how?! I couldn't logically and rationally fathom what I was seeing, my heart was pounding and furthermore, what were we going to do about it? Nothing had been said to Annie, so I thought 'first things first'. I explained exactly what I could see to Annie. She was naturally upset and frightened, she cried 'Am I pushing wrong?!'

I gave her reassurance, I told her she hadn't done anything wrong and this was an unforeseen and very rare occurrence. I was thinking that I had only ever seen this phenomenon in photographs. A small trickle of blood had been seen coming from the anus prior to the head suddenly becoming visible. I was told there hadn't been any time for an intervention to slow this process down. It seemed that the muscles of the perineum had torn from within as the baby moved down into the birth canal (Cortes, 2011).

At this point, Annie was still in the pool. I asked her to try not to push and for her to get out of the pool to review the situation on the bed with better access and a full view of the perineum.

I felt, although the warm water was soothing Annie's perineal tissue, that it would now be wise to leave the pool to manage the potential for heavy bleeding due to this extensive perineal trauma.

I asked for the obstetric team to be called, requesting an urgent medical review. We needed expert advice on this matter. Mick and I continued to help Annie out of the pool. I gently dried her and assisted her to the bed. Her contractions seemed to have come to a halt. I was thinking that the level of fear and anxiety may have caused an adrenaline rush, and that this in turn affected the natural rhythm of her contractions (Haines et al., 2012). I continued to listen to the foetal heart rate as per guidelines for the second stage (NICE, 2017c). Annie laid down in a semi-recumbent position, and I explained that I needed to place her legs into lithotomy.

As soon as I looked at the perineum, I knew exactly what I needed to do. Finally, I had a plan! I spoke with Annie in a calm but clear manner, informing her that I recommended performing an episiotomy as she pushed with the next contraction to try to minimise the risk of further, uncontrolled tearing. I used local anaesthetic to infiltrate the perineum. Annie wanted to know if her baby was okay. I reassured her that as the foetal heart rate was within normal range (NICE, 2017), it sounded as if her baby was coping well with events so far. My feeling was that once the episiotomy was performed, the baby would be born. All the while Mick was holding Annie's hand and helping Annie to focus on her breathing, saying 'everything is going to be okay, babe'.

I opened the delivery pack and prepared to perform the episiotomy. A few moments later, I was informed the consultant obstetrician was on her way. I was in a dilemma; should I wait for her to arrive or should I carry on?

I decided to carry on. I knew what was needed to be done and the sooner the better. A part of me really wanted someone else to be doing this, I was out of my comfort zone. The community midwife listened in to the foetal heart, did a set of observations on Annie, and got the room ready for the birth. I ran through the episiotomy technique in my head. Stay calm I was saying to myself.

I carefully infiltrated the paper-thin perineum with local anaesthetic. I heard the consultant enter the room and stand behind me; she introduced herself to both Annie and Mick. I asked her if she would like to take over, but she encouraged me to carry on. She was happy to just observe as she could see I was in control of the situation. I performed the episiotomy, guarding the anus as I did so (NICE, 2017b). The baby's head was born immediately, and restitution of the head took place pretty much straight away, adopting the ideal oblique position. Annie gave an involuntary push and the baby girl was born and cried spontaneously!

The baby was handed straight to Annie for skin to skin contact.

Annie had intramuscular Syntocinon administered with consent (NICE, 2017g); shortly afterwards the placenta and membranes were delivered. Annie's blood loss was minimal.

We carried on making Annie as comfortable as possible and keeping the ambience of the recent new birth at the forefront of the experience. Annie wanted to breastfeed her baby girl straight away, and with the baby skin to skin from birth, this was soon naturally initiated.

In view of the suspected anal trauma sustained during the birth, our plan was to move Annie to theatre for the repair of her perineum. Annie had a confirmed fourth-degree tear sutured in theatre by one of our consultants. A few days later she went home with no known complications.

Unexpected perineal trauma in the pool, buttonhole! Pat Hutson

Anastasia appeared to be working hard through her contractions on arrival and when she was eventually able to recover her breath, she felt ready to walk the few metres between the entrance door of our unit and the admission room. Once inside, she requested a vaginal examination to ascertain if she was in established labour (NICE, 2017h). I was happy to perform it and I found Anastasia's cervix to be 6 cm dilated and fully effaced. She had been experiencing strong and regular contractions for quite some hours before her arrival. We discussed pain relief options at length and Anastasia decided that although she had not previously considered using the pool, that she would like to try it, with the option of moving onto Entonox as and when she felt the need (NICE, 2017e). Her choices for pain relief were open, but she felt reluctant to have an epidural at this point, instead, she wanted to try the water, it seemed out of curiosity as much as anything else.

I ran the pool and checked the temperature to ensure it was optimal (Harper, 2014) and Anastasia got in. Within a short period of time she stated that the water was indeed helping and adopted a position she was comfortable in and established labour care was commenced (NICE, 2017f).

After a further 90 minutes, I noticed that the contractions had heightened in strength and Anastasia appeared to be bearing down with the occasional contraction. During the next hour, the bearing down became more frequent and I noticed external signs of descent of the presenting part, labial parting, and rectal flattening. These were all very indicative signs of full dilatation and so second stage labour care was commenced (NICE, 2017d). At this time, Anastasia became more mobile in the pool, moving from kneeling to sitting, trying to find a comfortable position. Whilst this was happening there appeared to be some blood loss, but due to the water movement it was unclear where this was originating from, therefore I requested that Anastasia vacated the pool for me to be able to accurately review the source of the bleeding. It was unclear whether it was from the perineum or vagina. Reluctantly, Anastasia agreed to leave the pool and made her way over to the bed.

Whilst she was lying on the bed, I noticed a small amount of blood draining which I thought was from Anastasia's vagina. It appeared to be a heavily blood-stained show. However, on further inspection, the perineum was becoming white and oozing with blood and this was in fact the source of the bleeding I had seen in the pool. I could see a large 'buttonhole', around the size of a ten pence coin, in the perineum. 'Button holing is when the top surface of skin between the Fourchette and the anal sphincter is stretched to an extent that the top layer of skin tears at the weakest point, it can also involve the rectovaginal septum' (Athanasiou et al., 2012). I described what I had seen to Anastasia and explained that the recommendation was for me to perform an episiotomy, to try to prevent the 'buttonhole' extending further. My thinking was that I would hopefully prevent Anastasia from having a resulting third- or fourth-degree tear by performing this manoeuvre (Collins, 2013; RCOG, 2015). The vertex was now visible and rapidly advancing. I summoned help into the room and prepared to perform the episiotomy. The baby's head was almost crowning by this point which made it difficult to administer the lidocaine prior to the episiotomy due to the perineum being stretched tightly over the presenting part. There was little space to insert my fingers in between the perineum and the baby's head but I persevered because I needed to first protect the baby's head from the needle used to infiltrate the lidocaine into the perineal skin (Gibbon, 2012) and I also needed to guard the head during the actual 'cut' of the episiotomy. I managed to both administer the lidocaine and perform a mediolateral episiotomy safely (NICE, 2017i). The head delivered with the next contraction and a healthy baby girl was delivered with the contraction after. The baby was a little 'shocked' but, once dried (Resuscitation Council (UK), 2016), let out a hearty cry within the first two minutes of life. Anastasia was delighted, although a little disappointed that she had not delivered her baby in the pool. When I inspected the perineum later, I noticed a large and complex second-degree tear, but a third- or fourth-degree tear had been avoided (NICE, 2017i).

A full debriefing was held with Anastasia the next day. The speed and complexity of the events made it difficult to discuss decisions contemporaneously. I explained the rationale for having managed the birth of Anastasia's baby out of the pool and thanked her for her cooperation during what must have been a very challenging time for her. She was delighted that she had been able to use the pool during most of her labour and felt it had made a huge difference and helped immensely.

A midwife's intuition and a mother's knowing: Sian Marie Barnard

Delphi had been labouring in the pool for several hours. The night shift midwife handed over to me and said that Delphi's contractions had been long and strong since just before midnight.

I could see instantly that Delphi was in strong established labour (NICE, 2017); she had a lean, athletic physique so it was easy to see the uterine muscle tense well with a contraction. During the breaks in between, she moved around freely in the pool, with a natural ease and agility. This was Delphi's second baby, her first child being only 18 months old. Her progress in labour had been adequate and with membranes still intact. The baby's head was found to be at −2 to the ischial spines but with position not determined. Shortly after the last examination, Delphi's membranes had ruptured, and clear liquor was reported as having 'gushed out' onto the incopad. As maternal and foetal observations were reported as normal following the spontaneous rupture of membranes (SROM; NICE, 2017j), I was told that Delphi got back in the water straight away. It was obvious that the pool had been a sanctuary for her.

Although, on the surface of it, the clinical picture appeared normal, I couldn't help but feel a slight sense of trepidation; okay, the rate of cervical dilatation had been satisfactory so far, from 4 cm to 6 cm cervical dilatation in four hours, but I couldn't help but wonder why strong, regular contractions had not heralded swifter progress given Delphi's parity and recent first, uncomplicated birth (NICE, 2017).

It was now approaching four hours from the last examination and Delphi unexpectedly looked up and told me she felt she couldn't do it any more ... she felt exhausted. This was quite a sudden proclamation, as it had only just been reported to me that previously she had been coping well. But Delphi had an overwhelming feeling of doubt and she just felt that 'she wasn't getting any closer'. This only confirmed my feelings of unease about Delphi's progress in labour. Given that she had been in the water, in the environment she so wanted to be, where reduced stress hormones and increased endorphins and oxytocin levels are a known benefit (Richmond, 2003), if anything, I had expected her labour to be efficient rather than prolonged.

I didn't feel her sentiments were due to the 'transition' of labour, her physical behaviour wasn't reflective of this at all. Delphi had been maximising on the soothing benefits of the water so beautifully, why now was she experiencing such a change of heart?!

My thoughts turned to offering a vaginal examination as it was due anyway, and this would enable me to 'feel' what was happening in terms of cervical dilatation and foetal position. I would then be able to formulate a proactive and informed plan of care that would best suit Delphi's needs. As she climbed out of the pool in preparation for me to perform the assessment on the bed, Delphi had another long, strong contraction causing a bloody mucousy show to appear at the introitus. I encouraged Delphi to try to pass urine and she managed to pass a normal void of dilute urine; two more long strong contractions whilst on the toilet brought no expulsive urges at all ... hmmm, this had me wondering.

Delphi climbed onto the bed and I performed the vaginal examination as agreed. I felt the cervix to be 8 cm dilated and fully effaced. This I was sure about; in terms of cervical dilatation, conservative but nevertheless normal progress (NICE, 2017f). I could feel the foetal skull against the rim of the cervix, but the station was still relatively high at −2 to the ischial spines; given the number of hours that Delphi had been contracting so strongly, I had expected more descent than this (Stables, 2000). However, the most surprising find was the large, fleshy prominence that met my fingers, protruding centrally through the cervix ... what was this? What was I feeling?! It didn't feel like caput, but more like the flesh of a cheek!

I was a little thrown to be honest. My abdominal palpation and Pinnard auscultation both confirmed a cephalic presentation, and on vaginal examination, I was sure I could feel the foetal skull and what I thought was a sagittal suture running in a transverse position above this. I was sure this baby was head down; but challenging my hypothesis was the presence of this anomaly that I couldn't explain as anything other than the flesh of a cheek. I just didn't understand. I questioned myself again, was this a cephalic presentation or is this a buttock I'm feeling … is this baby breech?!

Then I wondered if it could be cervix that had become trapped against the side of the foetal skull and subsequently become very swollen and oedematous? But no, I could feel a rim of cervix all the way round and much further back than this fleshy protrusion; it also seemed to be joined to a bone-like feature. Again, in my head I kept reiterating that I was sure I could feel the margin of the foetal skull and what I thought was a sagittal suture in a transverse position, a smooth, linear type indentation, with no defining features at either end of it. I was sure this baby was head down. But I just couldn't assimilate the fleshy prominence I was feeling with anything other than a breech presentation? Was I sure I wasn't missing something … genitalia or an anus, some defining feature that would make it clear?

This was not like anything I had ever felt before; I knew this was an unusual presentation, but which one?! I began to mentally place the pieces of the picture together: a very fleshy prominence centrally located, what felt like foetal skull and a possible suture line running transversely to this high in a 12 o'clock position in relation to Delphi's pubic bone. Then, it dawned on me – hang on – perhaps this is not buttock cheek I'm feeling, but facial cheek!

Once I'd had this realisation, the pieces of the puzzle fitted together, and it all made sense! I was 90% convinced that it was a face presentation, but unfortunately for Delphi, with this realisation came the likelihood that if I was right about this, then vaginal birth would be very unlikely (Sweet, 1997a). I needed to communicate this to Delphi in a sensitive, but very honest way.

Delphi had tolerated the examination so well, allowing me to carry on trying to fathom out what I was feeling under my fingertips; she breathed through the whole procedure admirably using the Entonox. I apologised to Delphi for the time it had taken me to perform the vaginal assessment; and went on to explain my findings to her (NICE, 2017j).

Delphi took the news well; she fully understood my explanation and she also told me she felt relieved to know the reason for the delay in her labour. She knew that the pool had afforded her the buoyancy and freedom of movement that are most conducive to a natural birth (Garland, 2011c), but she also knew she had hit a 'brick wall' that she was unable to knock down. It seemed that despite the liberating and enabling effects of the water, we had reached a labour impasse. What was so interesting was that our thoughts were in synchronisation in relation to this; mine based on midwifery intuition and Delphi's on her knowing as a mother.

Given my findings, I explained to Delphi what needed to happen next.

I requested an immediate ultrasound scan to confirm the foetal lie and presentation. Delphi's contractions had now all but disappeared due to the change in dynamics in her labour. It was almost as if the psychological disruption of this unexpected diagnosis was totally inhibiting her body's ability to make contractions (Meredith & Hugill, 2017). I wanted to ensure Delphi remained as calm as possible. Though it was obviously stressful for her, by talking to her, informing her, and reassuring her that her baby was not showing any signs of distress at all, I hoped to be able to keep the situation tolerable for Delphi. I emphasised that both her and baby were physically well, but also that this type of malpresentation would be likely to need obstetric intervention to enable the birth of the baby (Sweet, 1997a).

A consultant promptly arrived on the unit to perform the ultrasound scan. My findings were confirmed; the baby was indeed in a face presentation, with its neck extended at a 45° angle, and its cheek planted firmly and centrally in the os of the cervix. I had certainly never come across this before.

Delphi was promptly transferred to the obstetric unit following the scan and had an emergency caesarean section a little while later under very calm conditions. Her baby was unable to descend any further down into the birth canal due to the atypical inclination of its head compounding the complexity of the malpresentation. Both mother and baby were in perfect health following the surgery, with a bruised baby girl's cheek being the only clue that she had been in such an unusual and unexpected presentation!

Breech presentation and multi-professional teamwork: Pat Hutson

Barbara, a mother of two, arrived on our unit for intrapartum care. She had already been seen on the assessment unit by a colleague who indicated that her labour was established (NICE, 2017j). The pool was run in preparation for her arrival. As this was her third pregnancy, I was anticipating a speedy labour and birth. When I met her, she was unable to talk through her contractions and this led me to assume that she was indeed in established labour and progressing well (NICE, 2017j). I decided not to examine her, based on both her parity and her behaviour and helped her to get straight in the pool as was her wish.

Barbara's membranes ruptured soon after entering the pool. I immediately noticed that the water in the pool having previously been clear and transparent now appeared to be stained with what looked like meconium. The presence of meconium in the amniotic fluid is considered a deviation from normality and needs to be addressed. The presence of meconium in the liquor can be an indication of foetal compromise and needs to be treated as a potential emergency (NICE, 2017c), as there is the risk of aspiration as spontaneous breathing is initiated. As I looked more closely, I could see this was significant meconium, therefore I explained the need to exit the pool immediately to Barbara. I also advised transferring to the consultant-led unit, where electronic foetal monitoring should be commenced

(NICE, 2017c). As part of our protocol, the neonatal team would be summoned in advance, prior to the birth (NICE, 2017a). Barbara understood what I had said to her but was a little delayed in moving. I strongly advised her once again to leave the pool, quickly and calmly discussing the potential risks with her. She then vacated the pool promptly and I summoned help from my colleague. As I glanced down into the water again, I was suspicious at the amount of faeces present in the pool. It was difficult to assess because of the colour of the water. Barbara had begun to involuntarily push with her contractions prior to exiting the pool, so there were also some maternal faeces present in the water. I wondered if the fresh meconium I could see was a sign of breech presentation (Chadwick, 2002). Although this thought was now in my mind, I felt it was unlikely as Barbara's two previous babies had been born in a cephalic presentation. As she was walking towards the bed, she was sounding more and more expulsive and, on further inspection, the rectum appeared to be flattening out, a sign that the presenting part was descending (NICE, 2017d). All this had taken place in a very short time and Barbara had now begun to spontaneously push through the whole of her contraction. I still had doubts over the presentation, so it was my intention to perform a vaginal examination with Barbara's consent to confirm whether this baby was in a cephalic or breech presentation. My colleague appeared in the doorway to see what help I required. I calmly relayed my thoughts about the presentation and asked her to look into the pool to see what she could determine. She confirmed my thoughts that it was in fact toothpaste meconium at the bottom of the pool. Our suspicion about the baby being in the breech presentation was very strong, we needed to act quickly.

We needed to summon appropriate help and, as there appeared to be some labial parting, it was obvious that we did not have enough time to safely perform a vaginal assessment or transfer Barbara to the consultant-led unit (NICE, 2017d; Impey et al., 2017). In what I hoped was my calmest manner (I felt anything less than calm inside!), I explained to Barbara what was happening. I told her that we strongly suspected that the baby was breech, and about to be born. I was about to perform a vaginal examination when we saw something that did not look like a head descending. We explained that the obstetric and newborn teams would be attending in case help was needed. My colleague and I tried to reassure her as much as we could. We explained to the husband and mother what was happening, as they were becoming concerned with the activity in the room whilst not understanding what was occurring.

I tried to stay calm. I reassured Barbara that in order to best visualise descent of the presenting part, it would be wise for her to adopt an optimal all fours position on the bed (Evans, 2015; Impey et al., 2017). This she readily agreed and whilst she was moving onto her knees, the presenting part became fully visible. What was it, the bottom, a leg, a knee? At the same time, the obstetric and newborn emergency teams arrived and were greeted with a brief and succinct handover. The Resuscitaire was switched on in preparation should the baby need support when born. Barbara appeared to understand what was happening and was concentrating fully on the job she had in front of her.

Both teams had (thankfully) arrived quickly and the consultant obstetrician stood very calmly by my side and asked if I was confident to conduct the birth. She clearly stated that she would either support me or take the lead if either of us felt it became necessary. I felt reassured by the consultant's approach, which boosted my self-confidence with the task ahead. During the next ten minutes as the baby birthed itself, I remembered voicing my thoughts aloud by muttering buzz words like 'good cord profusion', 'nice cleft in the chest', and 'effective descent'. I was not sure who I was trying to reassure! Barbara's physical behaviour was textbook; she naturally moved into positions that are optimal for aiding a breech birth. Her body moved in conjunction with her baby, allowing the pelvis and the baby to work as one to optimise the descent (Evans, 2015). I recall feeling very anxious as the baby's bottom touched the bed, and I asked Barbara to lift her body up to facilitate the baby's descent. The consultant very quietly in my ear said, 'it's fine, just let her do what she needs to'. I will always remember her valuable advice. The baby delivered itself; arriving into the world with a lusty cry. At this point, I realised I had been holding my breath, I have no idea for how long. The gathered audience stared open mouthed at the beauty of what had just occurred, each one trying to relay the last few minutes to memory to be recalled on at a later stage if needed. I will be ever thankful to Dr Smith for trusting my ability to lead the delivery, and for allowing the woman to have a peaceful, calm breech birth with minimal intervention.

Unresponsive woman in the pool: Maria Paz Miranda

Tess was very excited about using the pool for her second birth. None of us knew by then the unusual course that the events would take that day. When we met her (I was working with a midwifery student that day), she had been enjoying the pool for the last three hours. Her first baby was born abroad, five years ago, where it was unheard of to use water in childbirth. She told us that labour was medicalised over there, and almost every woman, in her understanding of things, had an epidural at the beginning of labour. However, her husband wasn't very excited, and he expressed his concerns about the safety of his baby. He asked about electronic monitoring, something that he was expecting to happen. We discussed the indications of it and how in his wife's case, it wasn't recommended since she was healthy and carrying a low-risk pregnancy (NICE, 2017c). We showed him how we perform intermittent auscultation (IA), trying to reassure him as much as we could (RCM, 2012a and b; NICE, 2017c). Despite her husband's scepticism, Tess insisted on using the pool for her labour and birth.

Another few hours passed without any apprehensions. I could see Tess navigating the first stage of labour remarkably well and approaching second stage, smoothly and totally in control of her body. Within the next hour, she volunteered to abandon the pool to use the toilet.

When she returned to the pool, her attitude had changed. She was not coping so well now. The walking towards the toilet, the position adopted when sitting upright, had triggered strong contractions (RCOG, 2009). She asked whether she could have some additional pain relief for the first time. We discussed the options available in our unit (NICE, 2017e; Allan & Warriner, 2011). Tess was not familiar with Entonox, inhalational analgesia widely used in the UK, (Jones et al., 2012) but she was willing to try it.

Tess found the Entonox extremely helpful as her contractions felt milder and shorter when using it. Things were changing rapidly. Bloody, mucousy vaginal discharge appeared whilst experiencing strong rectal pressure, making her push involuntarily. Within the next few minutes, the baby's head was seen.

The student and I become very excited about the imminent birth. The other midwife working that day was made aware that Tess was actively pushing for 20 minutes when the unexpected happened.

She went very quiet and stopped pushing. Her body suddenly went relaxed and she was not answering our questions, or any questions: she was unresponsive. The baby's head was crowning, about to be born, and Tess appeared to be unconscious.

In the calmest way possible, I asked the student to press the emergency buzzer whilst I moved quickly by Tess's side and gently held her head out of the water. I looked at her husband and quickly explained what I thought was happening. Tess was in a state that I could not describe. Her eyes were half closed, and her body did not have any tone, but to my surprise, her respiratory rate and her pulse were normal. Foetal heart rate was 120 bpm and I did not hear any decelerations in those 20 seconds that I managed to listen in before my colleagues arrived ready to help!

'Tess is unresponsive, and we need to evacuate the pool. The baby's head is crowning, please call the emergency obstetric team and neonatal team to attend' I stated, feeling the pressure rising. The local emergency procedure was activated. A team of obstetrics doctors, an anaesthetist, the neonatal team, and the maternity bleep holder would be arriving within the next few minutes. The husband was warned.

Before the arrival of the emergency team, the six of us took on the task of the evacuating the pool using the net specially designed for this type of emergency. Four days before, in a quiet day in our unit, we had a practice situation of evacuating the pool. I was the woman in the water in our little exercise! Every manoeuvre was fresh in my memory.

One member of the team got the net out of the cupboard; simultaneously, two other members of the team disconnected our electric bed, moved it to the pool, levelled it to the same height of the pool, and removed the end of the obstetric bed. The net was already in place under Tess's body, including her head and pelvis. These manoeuvres took only one or two minutes, with three members of the team at each side of the pool, holding the net by the specifically designed handles (I was checking her perineum, the head was still crowning, it did not move!). 'On my count I said: one, two and three' and Tess's unresponsive body was lifted out of the pool and onto the bed.

Within the next few seconds, the foetal heart rate was auscultated, it was 90 bpm and maternal pulse was 70 bpm. My colleague had everything ready for an episiotomy to facilitate the birth of the head. I started to rub up a contraction, hoping that it would trigger a contraction strong enough to deliver the baby's head on its own, in view of an unresponsive mother unable to push. I was not successful in my attempt to generate a contraction … an episiotomy was my last alternative! (NICE, 2017b).

The other midwives had started maternal observations every five minutes using an electronic device. They were normal. During the process of evacuation, we kept talking to Tess, but she did not respond, and her body did not have any tone. I turned over to see whether I could speak with her husband to explain that I needed to perform an episiotomy. He was pale and answered me very quickly: 'please do whatever you need to do, but do it now'.

I was assessing the perineum for local infiltration when we saw Tess reacting to my touch. She seized the arm of a midwife and pushed as the emergency team entered the room. When they saw the head being born, they waited in a corner expectantly.

With the next push, the baby's body was born. It had good tone, but it was blue and not breathing properly. The neonatal doctor was next to me, giving me gentle guidance: 'wait, give the baby the time to recover' she said whilst the baby heart rate was auscultated. The rate was increasing. We positioned the head in a neutral position to facilitate the opening of the airways. The neonatal doctor, part of the emergency team in our hospital, had been by my side, observing, assessing. We decided to leave the umbilical cord intact to give the baby the chance to benefit from the extra blood present in the cord (Wylie et al., 2015). Fifty seconds later, the heartbeat was increasing rapidly, and then the baby cried, alleviating the anxiety of all of us (Michie, 1999). I felt unbelievable relief. After being sure that mother and baby were stable and well, the emergency team left, as perplexed as I was.

Tess had no recollection of what had happened to her.

After a lengthy debriefing session, we offered a strong coffee to an overwhelmed husband, who, at some point, abandoned the room to cry without been seen by his wife. The family stayed together in one of our postnatal rooms, where they could rest and try to overcome what they just had endured.

As a team, we sat for a few minutes to reflect on what just happened. I felt relieved that mother and baby were in good condition, despite the unusual circumstances of her birth.

A snapped cord! Sian Marie Barnard

At exactly 42 weeks of gestation, Ruby was due for induction of labour. She was so relieved when in the early hours of the morning that she was due to attend the induction of labour suite, her labour started spontaneously. Ruby was admitted to our unit, with a cervical dilatation of 3 cm, contracting strongly and regularly.

I walked into the room to meet Ruby, who was kneeling on the birthing couch, working hard at breathing through a long, strong contraction. I glanced at her birthing plan and read that it was Ruby's main wish to use water for labour (she described herself as a 'water baby'). I could see Ruby was in established labour (NICE, 2017) and finding the contractions difficult to manage, so this seemed the perfect time to mention using the pool. 'I'd love that' she said, but Ruby had a concern about waterbirth that was troubling her. Although she felt using water for labour was a totally natural option for her, she was very worried that if her baby was born underwater, he could be at risk. 'We're not amphibians' she said, 'Will he be ok?'

This was my perfect opportunity to allay her fears. I explained how her baby would be born from one aquatic existence to another; where the 'diving reflex' plays the key role in ensuring the baby doesn't take a breath underwater. I explained that this reflex closes structures in the baby's throat that will prevent fluid passing into the baby's lungs (Johnson, 1996). I could instantly see Ruby was fascinated and so relieved to hear this. As delayed cord clamping was also in her birth plan, I went on to discuss the relevance of this in relation to the continued cessation of breathing under the water (Wylie et al., 2016). I also explained how additional factors such as reduced gravity, appropriate water temperature, and the 'quietness' of birth underwater help to ensure breathing mechanisms are not triggered until the baby leaves the water (Garland, 2011b). Having heard all this, Ruby's mind was made up. With a new-found confidence, she now wanted to give birth in the pool! We formulated a plan of care between us. That was for her to enjoy the water, for me to perform observations as per guidelines, and to offer a vaginal examination in four hours to assess progress (NICE, 2017). This was a mutually agreed birth plan as Ruby and I were thinking synergistically, there was a meeting of minds and a lovely connection between us.

As soon as Ruby put one foot into the water, she smiled. As she sat down on the ledge of the pool, and even with her abdomen only half emerged, she said 'Ok, now I can do it, this is just what I wanted, thank you'.

Over the next few hours, labour went on to progress nicely. Three hours after she had entered the pool, I noticed Ruby's contractions were making her sound slightly expulsive. Without any commotion or fuss, she started to bear down in response to the pressure she was feeling with a naturalness and acceptance that was intriguing. She didn't seem disturbed by this sensation, but instead rather nonchalantly asked 'is it alright if it makes me poo in the water?' I thought this was so endearing and replied, 'If you feel you need to, yes!'

I could see bloody mucous show on the bottom of the pool and more at the introitus. I hadn't performed a vaginal examination, but I didn't need to straight away. I felt I would simply wait and see how Ruby behaved over the next half an hour. She was calm and acting instinctively, nothing more. Maternal and foetal observations were reassuring – all good I thought.

Three more contractions came and went without incident, then with the next, Ruby opened her eyes widely, stared into my eyes, and told me she now needed to push. 'Okay', I said, 'that's fine, but try to breathe through it if you can'. Initially, Ruby did just try breath the contraction away, but the overwhelming pressure she felt was too great; she let out a cry and gave a push down. As she did this, I could see the first glimpse of vertex appear. Amazing! This was extremely positive. 'Well done darling!' I said, 'I can just see the top of your baby's head!'

I was really pleased for Ruby; she had done so well. She had no intention of leaving the water now either; she was keen to have the waterbirth we had discussed earlier. Sure enough, the baby's head approached, crowning with the following contractions. The perineum looked to be stretching up beautifully. I called for a second midwife to assist me and scribe. With the next surge of pressure, the head was born. Ruby gathered her breath, and as the next contraction built, then she pushed steadily again. The posterior shoulder appeared first, then the anterior, it was almost as if the baby was 'shrugging' its shoulders free. There was a slight pause of only a few seconds then with another push the baby's body was born to the level of its lower stomach. The contraction had not fully passed, so I said to Ruby, 'Just give another little push, your baby's nearly out'. Looking down into the water, I noticed the cord was slightly pulling at the umbilicus.

Ruby pushed again, and the rest of the baby's body was born, but the cord was pulling more tightly at the umbilicus and was also taught in between this baby boy's legs. Because of an apparently short cord, the baby was tethered under the water for the first few moments. I was happy with his condition as he was pink and toned. I reassured Ruby that her baby was fine, but encouraged her to lift her bottom up in order to relieve the tension in the cord and enable me to bring him to the surface of the water. With this, Ruby panicked, leant forwards and took hold of the baby; hastily pulling him up towards her chest. I tried to steady the baby's ascent from the water, but as the traction on the cord continued, I saw the baby's body 'jerk' as he emerged from the water: the cord had snapped!

The uterine end of the cord recoiled under the water, retracting back in towards the introitus, seeping with blood as it did so. The baby cried immediately once in Ruby's arms. I looked to see if his cord was bleeding, or if there were any signs of blood loss from the umbilicus, but there were none to be seen. The remaining piece of cord still attached to the baby was already pale and redundant. It seemed as if the shock of the cord snapping had caused it to spasm; thus, the blood supply flowing through it had ceased (Morrin, 1997b). As luck would have it, the breakage had occurred leaving about 10 cm of cord proud of the umbilicus, so despite the baby's flailing limbs, I was quickly and easily able to apply the cord clamp!

The second midwife supported Ruby with holding the baby, whilst I quickly grasped the uterine end of the cord under the water and secured it with a cord clamp. I then breathed a sigh of relief, both ends of the cord were now secured! I gave oxytocic with consent (NICE, 2017g), estimating that only about 200 mL of blood was lost from the maternal end of the cord prior to clamping. With no concerning blood loss from either party, I was happy to proceed with calmly assisting Ruby out of the pool to manage the third stage of labour.

I asked the second midwife to perform an initial set of observations on the baby which were all within normal range (Wylie et al., 2016). Initial assessment of the baby led me to believe he had not been compromised by this event at all, but I asked the second midwife to request an immediate paediatric review considering the unusual circumstances. The second midwife and I both gave the baby an Apgar score of 10 at one minute from birth and 10 at five minutes from birth respectively (NICE, 2017a)

The paediatrician soon arrived and went on to perform a full assessment of the baby's wellbeing; she also gave the baby an Apgar score of 10 at ten minutes following the birth (NICE, 2017a), commenting that she also felt the baby had transitioned normally despite the cord having snapped unexpectedly (Wylie et al., 2016). The plan was to recommence skin to skin, encouraging the initiation of breastfeeding, and to continue observing the baby for the next 24 hours as a precaution. I thanked the paediatrician for coming, and she left with no concerns.

Ruby and I had a chat about things a little later. I felt it was important to debrief with her as she had said to me that she felt it was 'her fault' that the cord had snapped. I reassured her that this wasn't the case; I explained that although the cord was short and under tension, it was still highly unusual for it to break as it did. She seemed to feel better once she understood this. And there was another thing, Ruby's fears about a baby being born underwater were completely dispelled, she had witnessed a perfect demonstration of the diving reflex in action and was in no doubt that she would like another waterbirth for baby number two!

The early urges to push: Maria Paz Miranda

Sophie had experienced SROM, at home, before any contractions were felt. The couple had read and researched extensively about signs of labour, and consequently, when she found herself losing clear liquor all over her trousers, she realised that her membranes were broken. Very excited, she decided to call her community midwife for advice. The community midwife went to see Sophie at home and decided to perform a vaginal examination and found her cervix to be fully effaced and 4 cm dilated. Established labour was diagnosed (Hanley et al., 2016; NICE, 2017) and in view of the intensity and frequency of Sophie's contractions and the vaginal assessment findings, the community midwife suggested that she should go to the hospital for intrapartum care (RCM, 2012d).

On her arrival to our unit, Sophie expressed her wish to have a waterbirth, minimal intervention, and no pain relief unless she felt that she could not cope any more. Her wife led the conversation and gave me a detailed account of events: Sophie had been contracting for about four hours, starting an hour after her membranes broke. The contractions had increased in strength and length and Sophie told me that their intensity was increasing. She also felt that, even though she had read as much as she could about labour, she was feeling scared and anxious about her ability to cope with the intensity of the pain. I tried to reassure her as much as I could; she seemed to be a very strong young woman, loved and supported by her wife and it was easy to talk to her. We discussed the different stages of labour in depth, its progression and how the perception of pain and the release of endorphins were part of the same process and how the comfort of the warm water could help her to cope better (Cluett & Burns, 2009). We discussed the pain relief options available in our unit, but Sophie told me that she was doing well, and she did not need any (Allan & Warriner, 2014).

I was fully aware that she had been vaginally examined three hours before her arrival to our unit, and not by me. As vaginal examinations are subjective, it is always the possibility that there was an incongruence in the findings. However, Sophie was coping well, and the contractions were strong and regular, and getting into the pool seemed the right thing to do. My plan was to observe Sophie's behaviour and intervene only if I considered that it was necessary to reshape my plan of care. She was glowing with the news of the pool. I felt that a good rapport was developing. She was looking at me in an assertive and resolute manner.

Once in the water she was happy, enjoying the relaxation provided by the warm water that she was anticipating. About 30 to 40 minutes later, she felt the urge to push. These urges were growing by the minute and Sophie was now pushing with her contractions. I wondered whether she had reached full dilatation. It was possible, why not? Women always surprise us with their progression in labour, we must never forget this. However, in this case, I was unsure, so I decided to wait and see what happened after the next few contractions. Her wife started to encourage her to push, which I was not entirely comfortable with. I wondered whether they were early urges to push, meaning that full dilatation of the cervix had not been reached, or if she was 10 cm dilated, ready to push. I needed to think very carefully. After a few minutes of internal deliberation, I decided to perform a vaginal examination to formulate a plan according to the potential findings (RCM, 2012a).

Sophie was fit and healthy so getting out of the pool was an easy task for her. She left the pool, emptied her bladder and told me that she was ready and agreeing with a vaginal assessment. She was eager to know how far into this labour she was. She felt ready. Her cervix was now 5 cm dilated and fully effaced; it was central, and the baby's head was −2 to the ischial spines, tightly applied to the very thin cervix. I did not feel skull sutures, so I was unable to define the position of the baby but on the abdominal palpation performed by me before the examination, it did not impress me as an occipital posterior position of the baby. The findings were reassuring in the sense that she was in established labour and progressing well. However, she had not reached the second stage yet (NICE, 2017d). Sophie felt disappointed about the findings. She was feeling a strong rectal pressure and she did not understand why she was feeling that way, why she was not in the second stage of labour, ready to push. We had a frank discussion about the findings and its repercussions. It took me a good deal of time, trying to reassure her and her wife. Sophie went back into the pool, without any delay, expectant of what to do next. I needed to think very carefully. We were in front of two potential opposite scenarios.

a. If we assumed that Sophie was still 5 cm dilated, it could easily be another four to five hours of involuntary pushing, a process that could have the potential negative effect of making Sophie and her baby completely exhausted (Cooke, 2010), and possibly unable to continue labouring without intervention. In my analysis and in the back of my mind, I could not forget that avoiding intervention was a strong part of Sophie's birth plan.

b. Sophie could have progressed fast and therefore she could be approaching the second stage, in which case birth was almost imminent and I needed to be prepared for a precipitate birth.

It was a difficult decision to make. Still, her physical signs were of a woman in first stage. She was not compromised by the painful contractions, she was dealing with the pain extremely well, it was the rectal pressure that she found very uncomfortable and distressing. I was not seeing any vaginal discharge in the water, the familiar flattening of the perineum was not evident, so I did not see signs of further descent of the baby's head. I did not have other means to confirm my suspicions, but I was almost certain that I was in the presence of a strong woman navigating the first stage of her labour, feeling the rectal pressure increasing by the minute that needed my help and guidance. I discussed the rationale behind my advice and potential plan which the couple was willing to listen to and then try.

My plan included using Entonox (inhalational analgesia) to enable her to focus on her breathing and in that way allow her to control the urges to push. This suggestion needed a lot of explaining and reassurance as she did not want any pain relief at that point. However, she understood my thinking and agreed with it. A second component of the plan was adopting lateral and all fours positions in the pool, instead of the upright ones. I explained to Sophie and her wife that these actions were aimed to control her breathing and avoid an upright position that, in my opinion, would help to reduce the rectal pressure and decrease the early urges to push (Hillan, 1999; Walsh, 2012c). Even though there is not solid evidence supporting the fact that these measures really help with the increased rectal pressure and early urges to push, Sophie was prepared to try them. It took her a great deal of persistence and strength. She kept changing positions, on her side, right and left; she was remarkable. Although it was hard for Sophie to control the urges to push some of the time, she was incredibly strong in her determination to do this. Her enthusiasm was contagious, and I was truly impressed by her resilience and strength.

After a few minutes using Entonox, I could see the big change that I was expecting so much. It was great, the early urges diminished considerably and almost disappeared. This meant that Sophie could continue with her labour without further intervention or disruption. Four hours later she changed again. She told me that this time, the pressure was different and unbearable and that she was feeling very frightened about the next step in her labour. In fact, she could not finish her sentence and looking at me, she gave a strong and uncontrollable push! We both knew that this time, it was different! As calm as I could, I suggested that she could introduce one of her fingers into the introitus and see whether she could feel anything. She looked at me saying that her baby's head was just there, 2–3 cm away from the introitus! One hour after this, with Sophie pushing well and following her unbearable natural urges this time, a healthy baby boy was born, in the pool, without any further delay or complication. I was extremely glad to realise that my plan, tailored for Sophie's circumstances, had worked and helped her to birth her son without any further intervention as she wanted.

Learning points

Unexpected events in labour and birth are always stressful for everyone. No matter how well prepared we think we are, an unexpected event is always a surprise, and most of the time the unknown catches us off guard. A well-structured team and early recognition of the event might mitigate the adverse effects of it. It is impossible to anticipate the character of the event and the reactions of the staff and families involved; therefore, a pre-established set of guidelines of how to deal with these situations is extremely difficult to formulate.

However, childbirth and unexpected events during this process will always continue to challenge our practice. We believe that sharing our experiences will contribute to a better understanding and management of these unusual events.

Preventive

- Attend regular skills and drills updates.
- Familiarise yourself with the Apgar scoring system for the assessment of neonatal wellbeing.
- Practice your emergencies procedures again and again … ideally with your team.
- Be sure that you know where your emergency equipment is located and that you know how to use it.
- Early recognition of the abnormality may help to minimise maternal and neonatal morbidity.

During the unexpected event

- Nobody is familiar with an unexpected event. Stay calm and state clearly what is happening in the room and explain clearly and concisely what you need.

- Do not delay the emergency call ... the more helping hands during an unexpected situation, the better.
- Consider handing over the leading role if you are not sure how to manage the emergency.
- In an emergency, recite the manoeuvres and actions aloud.
- Let your team know what you are thinking and doing, they always have useful suggestions.
- Effective communication skills are key – explain the rationale for your actions to the woman.
- Try to 'normalise' the environment as much as possible to help facilitate the continuation of normal physiological birth.
- Intuitive midwifery is invaluable – listen to your 'inner voice' if you have concerns.
- Apply basic midwifery interventions before progressing towards invasive measures when deviating from normality.

After the event

- Structured debriefing is necessary and valuable to families and staff involved in the unexpected event.
- Reflect on the event – this will enable learning and improvements in practice.

References

Allan, L. & Warriner, S., 2011. OUH, Maternity information leaflets. [Online] Available at: www.ouh.nhs.uk/patient-guide/leaflets/files/110811spires.pdf [Accessed 22 November 2017].

Allan, L. & Warriner, S., 2014. The spires midwifery led unit. [Online] Available at: www. ouh.nhs.uk/patient-guide/leaflets/files/110811spires.pdf [Accessed 12 July 2018].

Athanasiou, S., Mousiolis, A., Grigoriadis, T., & Antsaklis, A., 2012. Case report: postpartum traumatic rectal tear after normal vaginal delivery with an intact anal sphincter. [Online] Available at: www.ics.org/Abstracts/Publish/105/000871.pdf [Accessed 19 March 2018].

Burns, E., 2004. Water: what are we afraid of? *The Practising Midwife*, 7(10), 17.

Chadwick, J., 2002. Malpresentations and malpositions. In: M. Boyle, ed. *Emergencies Around Childbirth: A Handbook for Midwives*. Abingdon: Radcliffe Medical Press, p. 66.

Cluett, E. & Burns, E. 2009. Immersion in water in labour and birth. [Online] Available at: www.ncbi.nlm.nih.gov/pmc/articles/PMC3982045 [Accessed 12 December 2018].

Coad, J. & Dunstall, M., 2001. The transition to neonatal life. In: *Anatomy and Physiology for Midwives*. Edinburgh: Mosby, p. 327.

Collins, S. et al. 2013. *Oxford Handbook of Obstetrics and Gynaecology*, 3rd edition. Oxford: Oxford University Press.

Cooke, A. 2010. When will we change practice and stop directing pushing in labour? *British Journal of Midwifery*, 18, February 2010.

Cortes, E., 2011. Waterbirth and pelvic floor injury: a retrospective study and postal survey using ICIQ modular long form questionnaires. *European Journal of Obstetrics Gynaecology and Reproductive Biology*, 155(1), 27–30.

Evans, J. 2015. Turning breech upside down. *MIDIRS*, 25(3), 325–330.

Garland, D., 2011a. Accentuating normality. In: *Revisiting Waterbirth: An Attitude to Care*. Basingstoke: Palgrave Macmillan, pp. 49–53.

Garland, D., 2011b. Breathing. In: *Revisiting Waterbirth: An Attitude to Care*. Basingstoke: Palgrave Macmillan, pp. 105–129.

Garland, D., 2011c. Why water? In: *Revisiting Waterbirth: An Attitude to Care*. Basingstoke: Palgrave Macmillan, p. 25.

Gibbon, K., 2012. How to perform an episiotomy. *Midwives Magazine*, 5.

Haines, H. M., Robertson, C., & Pallant, J., 2012. The influence of women's fear, attitudes and beliefs of childbirth on mode and experience of birth. *BMC Pregnancy and Childbirth*, 55, 12.

Hanley, G. E., Munro, S., Greyson, D., Gross, M. M., Hundley, V., Spiby, H., & Janssen, P. A., 2016. BMC pregnancy and childbirth. [Online] Available at: https://bmcpregnancychildbirth.biomedcentral.com/articles/10.1186/s12884-016-0857-4 [Accessed 19 November 2017].

Harper, B., 2014. Birth, bath and beyond: the science and safety of water immersion during labour and birth. *The Journal of Perinatal Education*, 23(3), 124–134.

Hillan, E., 1999. *Mayes' Midwifery: A Textbook for Midwives: Physiology and Management of the Second Stage of Labour*, 13th edition. Edinburgh. Churchill Livingstone, p. 453.

Impey, L. W. M., Murphy, D. J., Griffiths, M., & Penna, L. K., on behalf of the Royal College of Obstetricians and Gynaecologists, 2017. Management of breech presentation. *BJOG*, 124, e151–e177. [Online] Available at: http://onlinelibrary.wiley.com/doi/10.1111/1471-0528.14465/epdf [Accessed 2 February 2018].

Johnson, P., 1996. Birth underwater-to breath or not to breath? *British Journal of Obstetrics & Gynaecology*, 103 (March), 202–8.

Jones, L., Othman, M., Dowswell, T., Alfirevic, Z., Gates, S., Newburn, M., Jordan, S., Lavender, T., & Neilson, J. P., 2012. Pain management for women in labour: an overview of systematic reviews. *Cochrane Database of Systematic Reviews* [Online] Available at: http://onlinelibrary.wiley.com/doi/10.1002/14651858.CD009234.pub2/full#pdf-section [Accessed 4 November 2017].

Kitzinger, S. 2000. *Rediscovering Birth*, 1st edition. London: A Little Brown Book.

Meredith, D. & Hugill, K., 2017. Motivations and influences acting on women choosing homebirth: seeking a 'cwtch' birth setting. *British Journal of Midwifery*, 25(1), 10–14.

Michie, M. M., 1999. Baby at birth, assessment of the baby's condition. In: Bennett, Ruth V., & Brown, Linda K., ed. *Myles' Midwifery: A Textbook for Midwives*, 13th edition. Edinburgh: Churchill Livingstone, pp. 672–673.

Morrin, N., 1997a. Midwifery care in the second stage of labour. In: B. Sweet, ed. *Mayes' Midwifery: A Textbook for Midwives*. Edinburgh: Bailliere Tindall, pp. 385–402.

Morrin, N., 1997b. Midwifery care in the third stage of labour. In: B. Sweet & D. Tiran, eds. *Mayes' Midwifery: A Textbook for Midwives*. Edinburgh: Bailliere Tindall, pp. 403–417.

NICE, 2012. Neonatal infection (early onset): antibiotics for prevention and treatment. NICE Guidelines [CG149]. [Online] Available at: www.nice.org.uk/guidance/cg149/chapter/1-Guidance#riskfactors-for-infection-and-clinical-indicators-of-possible-infection-2 [Accessed 19 November 2017].

NICE, 2014. Pain relief. [Online] Available at: https://pathways.nice.org.uk/pathways/intrapartum-care/pain-relief-in-labour#content=view-node%3Anodes-pain-relieving-strategies [Accessed 16 February 2018].

NICE, 2017. Intrapartum care for healthy women and babies. NICE Guidelines [CG190] First stage of labour. [Online] Available at: www.nice.org.uk/guidance/cg190/chapter/Recommendations#first-stage-of-labour [Accessed 12 October 2018].

NICE, 2017a. Intrapartum care for healthy women and babies. NICE Guidelines [CG190]. Care of the new born baby. [Online] Available at: www.nice.org.uk/guidance/cg190/chapter/Recommendations#care-of-the-newborn-baby [Accessed 24 April 2018].

NICE, 2017b. Intrapartum care for healthy women and babies. NICE Guidelines [CG190]. Intrapartum interventions to reduce perineal trauma. [Online] Available at: www.nice.org.uk/guidance/cg190/chapter/Recommendations#second-stage-of-labour [Accessed 2 September 2018].

NICE, 2017c. Fetal monitoring. [Online] Available at: https://pathways.nice.org.uk/pathways/intrapartum-care#path=view%3A/pathways/intrapartum-care/fetal-monitoring-during-labour.xml&content=view-node%3Anodes-when-to-offer-continuous-cardiotocography-and-telemetry [Accessed 15 December 2017].

NICE, 2017d. Intrapartum care for healthy women and babies. NICE Guidelines [CG190]. Second stage of labour. [Online] Available at: www.nice.org.uk/guidance/cg190/chapter/Recommendations#second-stage-of-labour [Accessed 12 February 2018].

NICE, 2017e. Intrapartum care for healthy women and babies. NICE Guidelines [CG190]. Pain relieving strategies. [Online] Available at: www.nice.org.uk/guidance/cg190/chapter/Recommendations#pain-relief-in-labour-nonregional [Accessed 19 March 2018].

NICE, 2017f. Intrapartum care for healthy women and babies. NICE Guidelines [CG190]. Care throughout labour. [Online] Available at: www.nice.org.uk/guidance/cg190/chapter/Recommendations#care-throughout-labour [Accessed 4 October 2017].

NICE, 2017g. Intrapartum care for healthy women and babies. NICE Guidelines [CG190]. Third stage of labour. [Online] Available at: www.nice.org.uk/guidance/cg190/chapter/Recommendations#third-stage-of-labour [Accessed 16 March 2018].

NICE, 2017h. Intrapartum care for healthy women and babies. NICE Guidelines [CG190]. Initial assessment. [Online] Available at: https://www.nice.org.uk/guidance/cg190/chapter/Recommendations#initial-assessment [Accessed 12 January 2018].

NICE, 2017i. Intrapartum care for healthy women and babies. NICE Guidelines [CG190]. Intrapartum interventions to reduce perineal trauma. [Online] Available at: www.nice.org.uk/guidance/cg190/chapter/Recommendations#second-stage-of-labour [Accessed 2 September 2018].

NICE, 2017j. Intrapartum care for healthy women and babies. NICE Guidelines [CG190]. Observations during the established first stage. [Online] Available at: www.nice.org.uk/guidance/cg190/chapter/recommendations#first-stage-of-labour [Accessed 16 March 2018].

NMC, 2015. *The Code: Standards of Conduct, Performance and Conduct for Nurses and Midwives*. London: NMC.

RCM, 2012a. Evidence based guidelines for midwifery-led care in labour. Assessing progress in labour, P 3. [Online] Available at: www.rcm.org.uk/sites/default/files/Assessing%20Progress%20in%20Labour.pdf [Accessed 12 December 2017].

RCM, 2012b. Evidence based guidelines for midwifery-led care in labour. Intermittent auscultation. [Online] Available at: www.rcm.org.uk/sites/default/files/Intermittent%20Auscultation%20%28IA%29_0.pdf [Accessed 12 December 2017].

RCM, 2012c. Evidence based guidelines for midwifery-led care in labour. Supporting women in labour. [Online] Available at: www.rcm.org.uk/sites/default/files/ Supporting%20Women%20in%20Labour_1.pdf [Accessed 28 November 2017].

RCM, 2012d. The Royal College of Midwives. Evidence based guidelines for midwifery-led care in labour. [Online] Available at: www.rcm.org.uk/sites/default/files/Introduction. pdf [Accessed 11 November 2017].

RCOG, 2009. RCOG statement on maternal position during the first stage of labour. [Online] Available at: www.rcog.org.uk/en/news/rcog-statement-on-maternal-position-during-the-first-stage-of-labour/ [Accessed 12 November 2017].

RCOG, 2015. The management of third- and fourth degree tears. [Online] Available at: https://www.rcog.org.uk/globalassets/documents/guidelines/gtg-29.pdf [Accessed 2 March 2018].

RCOG, 2017. Group B streptococcal disease, early-onset green-top guideline No. 36. [Online] Available at: www.rcog.org.uk/en/guidelines-research-services/guidelines/ gtg36/ [Accessed 5 December 2018].

Resuscitation Council (UK), 2016. *New Born Life Support*, 4th edition. London: Resuscitation Council (UK).

Richmond, H., 2003. Women's experience of waterbirth. *The Practicing Midwife*, March 6(3), 26–31.

Simpson, C., 1997. Respiratory disorders of the neonate. In: B. Sweet, ed. *Mayes' Midwifery: A Textbook for Midwives*. Edinburgh: Bailliere Tindall, pp. 860–867.

Stables, D., 2000. Malposition and cephalic malpresentations. In: *Physiology in Childbearing with Anatomy and Related Biosciences*. Edinburgh: Bailliere Tindall, pp. 520–521.

Sweet, B., 1997a. Malpresentations. In: B. Sweet & D. Tiran, eds. *Mayes' Midwifery: A Textbook for Midwives*, 12th edition. Edinburgh: Bailliere Tindall, pp. 651–654.

Sweet, B., 1997b. Malpositions of the fetal head. In: B. Sweet & D. Tiran, eds. *Mayes' Midwifery: A Textbook for Midwives*, 12th edition. Edinburgh: Bailliere Tindall, pp. 631–636.

Sweet, B., 1997c. Midwifery Care in the second stage of labour. In: *Mayes Midwifery: A Textbook for Midwives*, 12th edition. Edinburgh: Bailliere Tindall, pp. 631–636.

Walsh, D., 2012a. Rhythms in the third stage of labour. In: *Evidence and Skills for Normal Labour and Birth A Guide for Midwives*. Abingdon: Routledge, pp. 138–139.

Walsh, D., 2012b. Water immersion and waterbirth. In: *Normal Labour and Birth A Guide for Midwives*. Abingdon: Routledge, p. 145.

Walsh, D., 2012c. Rhythms in the second stage of labour. In: *Evidence and Skills for Normal Labour and Birth: A Guide for Midwives*. Abingdon: Routledge, pp. 110–111.

Wylie, J., Ainsworth, S., & Tinnion, R., 2015. Resuscitation Council (UK). Resuscitation and support of transition of babies at birth. Introduction. [Online] Available at: www. resus.org.uk/resuscitation-guidelines/resuscitation-and-support-oftransition-of-babies-at-birth/#changes [Accessed 14 December 2017].

Wylie, S., Ainsworth, S., & Tinnion, R., 2016. Physiology of transition at birth and perinatal hypoxia. In: Resuscitation Council (UK). *Newborn Life Support*, 4th edition. London: Resuscitation Council UK, pp. 11–24 .

Index